Praise for *The Body Fat Solution*

"Offering the opposite of a quick fix, Venuto is honest about the effort it takes to drop a significant number of pounds. This is the book for women ready to tackle long-term weight loss."

—Polly Brewster, *O: The Oprah Magazine*

"Venuto gets at all the physical, psychological, and even sociological aspects of overeating, outlining a program of mental, cardio, and strength training, stressing accountability and self-control. Nothing fluffy about this book: just well-founded scientific research and clearly illustrated direction."

—Raya Kuzyk, media editor, *Library Journal*

"Read this book—if you want to lose weight, improve your body and your health, and keep up these improvements for life. Tom Venuto gives it to you straight, basing his program on solid science and common sense. You will come away with a new feeling of inspiration and a new action plan to get you started and keep you on track to help you reach your goals—and then beyond."

—Judith S. Beck, Ph.D., author of *The Complete Beck Diet for Life*;
Director, Beck Institute for Cognitive Therapy and Research;
and research associate professor for psychology
in psychiatry, University of Pennsylvania

"At last, easy, concise, no excuses: get skinny—this is the guide. Great work, Tom!"

—Richard Bandler, co-developer of NLP (neuro-linguistic programming)
and author of *Get the Life You Want*

"Tom Venuto's *Body Fat Solution* is one of the most important books on health, happiness, and physical well-being. With this fast-moving, easily usable series of methods and techniques, you learn how to enjoy superb physical fitness, achieve your ideal weight, and feel terrific about yourself, both emotionally and spiritually."

—Brian Tracy, motivational speaker and author of *Reinvention*

"In 2003, Tom Venuto changed the fat-loss world with his e-book *Burn the Fat, Feed the Muscle*. In 2008 he's done it again, with *The Body Fat Solution*. The world's expert on fat loss speaks—I listen. I've often said that fat loss doesn't start with an exercise program, a diet, or a supplement; it starts with a mind-set shift. That mind-set shift begins with Tom's new book. If you want to change your body, you need to change your mind. And to do that, you need Tom Venuto."

—Alwyn Cosgrove, coauthor of *The New Rules of Lifting*
and *The New Rules of Lifting for Women*

"*The Body Fat Solution* hits the nail on the head. After working in the weight-loss arena for years, I've learned it's difficult to find a book that truly spells out what it takes to lose weight permanently. It's not a gimmick, it's not a quick fix, but it surely is a solution!"

—Christopher R. Mohr, Ph.D., R.D., cofounder of Mohr Results, Inc.

"*The Body Fat Solution* is going to change the paradigm in terms of weight loss. Most people believe that it's a particular program that will be the answer, but as Tom covers in his book, it's more about what gets each of us to follow *any* program—the behavioral factors that are so critical in achieving success. His new book perfectly addresses the science of exercise and behaviorial psychology together, a powerful combination!"

—Steve Yu, producer of *Inspired: The Movie*

"*The Body Fat Solution* provides solutions for regular people who live with stress, a shortage of time, and emotional eating habits, and who lack motivation. Through reading and implementing this book, readers will be able to promote successful thinking, stop bingeing and self-sabotaging behavior, lose fat, increase muscle, eat delicious foods, become motivated, quit dieting, increase metabolism, break the fat-loss plateau, lose those last few pounds, and develop a positive social network."

—Kelly Jad'on, book reviewer and syndicated health columnist, *Basil & Spice*

"Look for *The Body Fat Solution* to become the best seller of the new year."

—Jim Foster, www.diet-blog.com

"Thank you so much for writing *The Body Fat Solution*. After reading the book, I decided to download the audio version and listen to it over and over again. The principles you shared have helped me to help my clients finally realize their self-limiting behaviors and have brought an awareness of destructive habits that was missing in the fitness marketplace. I highly recommend this book, an instant classic!"

—Jimi Varner, personal trainer

"*The Body Fat Solution* outlines all of the necessary tactics to tackle intangible influences on our nutrition and exercise plans. The most insightful and logical nutrition and exercise program I have ever seen. Everything you need to know . . . it's all there. Very motivational and very doable!"

—Wade Weatherington, M.D., FAAP

"*The Body Fat Solution* is an amazing, life-changing book. When you are ready, this is the book to read. I found Tom Venuto's book in my time of need. We all know what to do, but Tom gives us the how, the whys, and the science behind the facts. Somehow, understanding the whys helps so much more than someone just telling me what to eat or not to eat. This book should be mandatory reading in every health class across the United States. This would help solve the obesity crisis in America."

—John D. Kovac, M.D.

THE
BODY
FAT
SOLUTION

THE BODY FAT SOLUTION

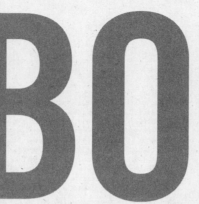
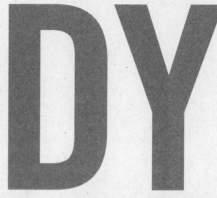

Five Principles for **Burning** Fat, **Building** Lean Muscles, **Ending** Emotional Eating, and **Maintaining** Your Perfect Weight

TOM VENUTO

AVERY
a member of
Penguin Group (USA) Inc.
New York

Published by the Penguin Group

Penguin Group (USA) Inc., 375 Hudson Street, New York, New York 10014, USA •
Penguin Group (Canada), 90 Eglinton Avenue East, Suite 700, Toronto, Ontario M4P 2Y3,
Canada (a division of Pearson Penguin Canada Inc.) • Penguin Books Ltd, 80 Strand, London WC2R 0RL, England •
Penguin Ireland, 25 St Stephen's Green, Dublin 2, Ireland (a division of Penguin Books Ltd) •
Penguin Group (Australia), 250 Camberwell Road, Camberwell, Victoria 3124, Australia
(a division of Pearson Australia Group Pty Ltd) • Penguin Books India Pvt Ltd,
11 Community Centre, Panchsheel Park, New Delhi–110 017, India •
Penguin Group (NZ), 67 Apollo Drive, Rosedale, North Shore 0632, New Zealand
(a division of Pearson New Zealand Ltd) • Penguin Books (South Africa) (Pty) Ltd,
24 Sturdee Avenue, Rosebank, Johannesburg 2196, South Africa

Penguin Books Ltd, Registered Offices: 80 Strand, London WC2R 0RL, England

First trade paperback edition 2009
Copyright © 2009 by Tom Venuto

Photographs by Jason Jaskot

Most Avery books are available at special quantity discounts for bulk purchase for sales promotions, premiums, fund-raising, and educational needs. Special books or book excerpts also can be created to fit specific needs. For details, write Penguin Group (USA) Inc. Special Markets, 375 Hudson Street, New York, NY 10014.

Library of Congress Cataloging-in-Publication Data

Venuto, Tom.
The body fat solution : five principles for burning fat, building lean muscles, ending emotional eating,
and maintaining your perfect weight / Tom Venuto.
p.   cm.
ISBN 978-1-58333-373-0
1. Weight loss.   2. Reducing exercises.   3. Nutrition—Psychological aspects.   I. Title.
RM222.2V46   2009b   2009035955
613.7'12—dc22

Printed in the United States of America
1   3   5   7   9   10   8   6   4   2

BOOK DESIGN BY TANYA MAIBORODA

Acknowledgments

Writing a book might seem to be a solo endeavor, but although you have to do it alone, you can't do it by yourself. I'm grateful to all those who supported, influenced, and believed in me during the journey to take this book from dream to reality.

First and foremost, I'd like to thank and acknowledge my agent, Stephen Barbara of the Donald Maass Literary Agency. Quite simply, *The Body Fat Solution* would not exist without you and your persistent efforts. You didn't just believe in this book, you believed in me. I'd also like to thank Megan Newman, Miriam Rich, and the team at Avery for believing in the integrity of the message in this book and helping bring it to the world . . . and thank you for your infinite patience.

To my mom and dad: thank you for your help, support, all the hours you let me bounce ideas off you, and, more important, for always encouraging me to pursue my dreams and be true to myself. And to my brother, Steve, thanks for the support. Can we go to Vegas now?

Some of the psychology and behavioral change principles in this program are based on Neuro-Linguistic Programming (NLP). I'd like to acknowledge Richard Bandler and John Grinder as the cofounders of this technology for personal change and modeling human excellence. Special thanks to Richard Bandler and John LaValle for making these teachings available through the

NLP society. Barbara Stepp—thank you for being a legendary coach and teacher. Thanks to Doug O'Brien, Jonathan Altfeld, and Robert Dilts for your excellent work on beliefs. To Pete Siegel, hypnotherapist, peak performance coach, and all-around human dynamo—thanks for the encouragement.

To the giants of the personal development industry: Jim Rohn, Brian Tracy, Bob Proctor, Mark Victor Hansen, Jack Canfield, Denis Waitley, Steven Covey, Tom Hopkins, Tony Robbins, the late Earl Nightingale, and the "Father of Motivation," Dr. Wayne Dyer. Thank you for doing what you do. Personal development has helped make me the person I am today. I hope that many more people discover that only by standing on the shoulders of giants can we see beyond our present horizons.

To Richie Smyth: everyone should have a trainer. Not everyone is lucky enough to have the best one, as I do. To Kyle Battis and John Sifferman: thanks for holding down the fort while I was in my writing cave. You guys rock. To Lee Howard: thanks for helping me polish up the first drafts of my manuscript. To Christian Dilalla for the cover shot and Jason Jaskot for the exercise photos. To our models, Liz and Joey, you were great!

I'm indebted to all the practitioners and researchers who are doing such fabulous work in the fields of nutrition, training, and the psychology of weight control today. Those who influenced this book especially include:

Dr. Brian Wansink, for the brilliant research on mindless eating; Dr. Judith Beck, for the superb work in cognitive psychology applied to weight loss; Dr. Charles Garfield, for the classic work on peak performance; Dr. John Bargh and Dr. Tanya Chartrand, for your insightful work on the unconscious mind; Barbara Rolls, Ph.D., for the clinical research and accessible writings on energy density; Rena Wing and Dr. James Hill, for the outstanding work with the National Weight Control Registry; Dr. John Berardi, for some of the best fat-loss and sports-nutrition information available today; Alwyn Cosgrove, for the excellent work on designing training programs for fat loss and for sharing it with other fitness professionals; and Ian King, for influencing many of my philosophies on strength training.

Finally, I thank the hundreds who gave me the privilege of being their personal trainer through the 1990s and early 2000s, and to the hundreds of thousands who have read my e-newsletters and supported me since I began as an Internet writer in 1999. I would not be here in print today had all of you not placed your faith in me as your trainer and coach for the first ten years of my career and as your source of Internet information for the last ten.

Contents

Part Two   The Five Principles

Part Three   Putting It All Together

Part Four   Appendices

THE
BODY
FAT
SOLUTION

Introduction

As an aspiring teenage bodybuilder in the mid-1980s, I was initiated into the world of body transformation. That's when I began learning a philosophy and methodology so effective for getting lean, I was ultimately able to achieve body fat as low as 3.7 percent while at my competition peak. To give you some idea of what that means, the average male has about 17 percent body fat and the average female has about 25 percent. If you want to see six-pack abs, you'll usually need to drop to under 10 percent body fat if you're male and down to about 15 percent or so if you're female.

Three percent is essential body fat in men, which is the amount necessary just to stay healthy. This means my body fat got so low, virtually no fat was left beneath my skin. People told me I looked like a walking anatomy chart. In bodybuilding vernacular, the word for that is "ripped." Mind you, I'm not naturally lean. Before I learned how to cut body fat, I'd never seen my abs. In fact, I was a slightly chubby freshman in high school, embarrassed to take my shirt off for swimming class. How things changed.

By my twenties, I became a multititle winner in bodybuilding and got so lean and muscular that many people thought I was taking steroids or fat-burning drugs. The truth is, I have never taken a banned or illegal performance-enhancing substance in my life. I developed my physique naturally with nutrient-dense food, a carefully controlled calorie intake, progressive resistance weight training, the right dose of cardio, a mind focused on well-formed goals, strong emotional drive, and a great support system of friends, training partners, and mentors.

I realized, of course, that most people had no interest in bodybuilding. Nevertheless, I was sure the type of nutrition programs I was using for fat reduction with such success could work for others even if they had more modest goals. So I compiled my fat-burning techniques into an organized system and began teaching them to others.

Since 1990, I've personally trained hundreds of people one-on-one in the gym. More than six hundred people graduated from my twelve-week "Burn the Fat" coaching program, which later became the basis of my first self-published e-book, *Burn the Fat, Feed the Muscle*. Since the Internet boom at the turn of the millennium, tens of thousands of men and women from more than 143 countries have used my Web-based fat-burning programs, hundreds of thousands have subscribed to my e-mail newsletters, and millions have visited my websites and blogs.

How Effective Does Your Fat-Burning Program Need to Be?

Under my guidance, men and women were cutting body fat like crazy, even when they'd been stuck for years with stubborn belly fat or diet-resistant lower-body flab. I've lost count of how many of my clients have joined my 100 Pounds Gone Club and more than one has shed over two hundred pounds. I also worked with people who weren't overweight. They started with average body fat levels, and I helped them reach the extreme leanness necessary for bodybuilding, fitness, figure, or before-and-after transformation contests.

Despite the fact that people of every size, shape, age, and background were succeeding using my advice, I noticed that something was missing. I seemed to attract a certain type of client, and most of them had a few things in common: they were all highly motivated, they all wanted to maximize their results, and they were all willing to do whatever it took to achieve their goals. These people were *serious*.

I'm not sure if it was my physical appearance, my "no shortcuts" work ethic, or my "no gimmicks" approach that drew these people to me. Maybe it was because my programs had their origin in the subculture of bodybuilders and fitness models, a fact many people found intriguing. On the other hand, it was very intimidating to others. My guess is that some people were thinking, "I'm not interested in gaining muscle," or "I don't need to be 'ripped.'"

When I started in the fitness business, it never would have dawned on me that a program could be too effective or too sophisticated. Truth be told, I was always looking for advanced diet tricks or some extra competitive edge to shed that final ounce of fat. In hindsight, I now see that the programs I prescribed may have been the most effective in the world, but they were like shooting a squirrel with a cannon! It's nice to have all that firepower, but it's overkill for the job.

My New Solution for Millions of "Regular People"

For a long time I believed that maximizing results depended on doing nutrition strictly by the numbers and also customizing those numbers for every individual. Ultimately, I realized the only thing necessary for most people to succeed was a handful of daily behavior changes and a shift in mind-set. I also learned I didn't have to explain all the mechanisms, only provide the action steps. You don't need to understand electricity to light your home, you only need to know how to flip the switch.

My new keyword became "simplicity." I grew convinced that by developing a simple new lifestyle program, I would be able to help, not tens of thousands of serious and already motivated fitness enthusiasts, but tens of millions of regular people to get the bodies of their dreams. I wanted to help people with common everyday challenges, such as high stress, lack of time, emotional eating, and sporadic motivation. I needed a solution with principles so simple that people would no longer ask, "Will it work for me?" but would instead say, "I can do that!"

By stepping outside my world of high-level physique transformation toward the wants, needs, and goals of ordinary "real people," I finally figured out how to create such a program: I worked backward. I started with the causes and traced them back to the solutions.

What's the *Real* Cause of the Body Fat Problem?

I could only succeed in reverse engineering a solution by understanding that body fat is a problem with multiple causes, including inactivity, diet, hormones, genetics, mental programming, emotions, environment, and social pressure. As diverse as they may seem, these factors all lead to one pivotal point in the causal chain: a calorie surplus.

If you have more body fat than you want, it's because you've been consuming more calories than you've been burning. Knowing this, however, doesn't tell you why you have a calorie surplus in the first place. I'm sure you've heard "Eat less and exercise more" hundreds of times, but following this advice alone didn't solve the problem, did it? *The Body Fat Solution* acknowledges calorie management as the key to body fat control, but at the same time it delves further to find the root causes of overeating and inactivity.

The explanations proposed for excess food intake and obesity are limitless and the debates about the best way to lose fat seem never ending. One reason why there's no consensus is because so many authorities on health, fitness, and weight control are heavily vested in their own theories and ideologies.

In the last few decades, when health and weight-loss experts have come across a new discovery in obesity research, they've often taken that one aspect of this multifaceted problem and created an entire program around it. One "evil culprit" is often blamed as the cause or one "magic bullet" praised as the cure or solution.

Though there are others too numerous to mention, examples include:

- All types of low-carbohydrate diets that drastically reduce sugar and carbs
- Low-glycemic-index diets that recommend specific types of carbs
- Low-fat diets that reduce intake of dietary fat
- Omega, Mediterranean, or fish-oil diets that increase consumption of essential fats
- Paleolithic diets that eliminate modern processed foods
- Metabolic typing or diets that prescribe macronutrient ratios (for example, the 40-30-30 diet)

- Inflammation (anti-inflammatory diet)
- pH balance (acid-alkaline diet)
- Detoxification diets to purge harmful substances from the body
- Hormones—insulin, growth hormone, leptin, thyroid, cortisol, and testosterone (there's a diet revolving around each one, believe it or not)

Each one of these approaches may contain important and scientifically valid information. Because there may be truth in all of them, readers seldom question their integrity or efficacy, nor should they, in most cases. What they should question is whether making *one* change in diet or targeting a single cause will solve a problem as complex as obesity. Unfortunately, it's the norm for a new or contrarian approach to take the spotlight—not because it's a breakthrough worthy of center stage, but because the marketplace demands and thrives on novelty.

Year after year, you've seen one "next big thing" after another, and yet you've usually been left disappointed each time. Every new diet seems to be based on a unique idea. Each sounds plausible. Some contain a thread of truth, but they all fall short if they contain only a single thread in a much larger tapestry. What's been missing in every case can be summed up in a single word: synergy. We've focused on isolated details, but missed the big picture of how all the pieces work together in real life for real people.

Why is there still a body fat problem today, and how do we solve it? I've devoted my adult life and career to studying these questions. Not only have I found answers, I've put them all together into a simple five-part formula that will work for millions of people, including you. It's a synergistic, total-life approach that addresses all of the true root causes of the body fat problem in every area of your life—physical, mental, emotional, and social. It's called the Body Fat Solution.

Whom This Book Is For

Recommendations and claims for fitness, weight loss, and especially for health must be put into context. I believe *The Body Fat Solution* can potentially help millions of people, but its approach is not for everyone.

First and foremost, *The Body Fat Solution* was written for men and women who are overweight. It's also for people who were previously overweight who want to maintain their ideal weight for the rest of their lives. This book is for the busy working person who doesn't have all day to spend in the gym or in the kitchen preparing complicated meals. It was not written for the full-time athlete, bodybuilder, fitness professional, or person with unlimited time to exercise.

The Body Fat Solution is for the layperson who wants simple explanations and practical action strategies to apply in daily life. This book is based on scientific research, but it was not written for the academic type who wants stoic reporting of all the latest studies.

The Body Fat Solution is strictly a fitness and fat-burning program. It's not for people with serious medical problems. By shedding excess body fat, many of your major health indicators are likely to improve dramatically. However, the exercise and nutrition suggestions in this program are not intended for clinical purposes. Always consult your physician, dietitian, or clinical nutritionist for advice before starting any exercise or nutrition program.

What You Can Expect from the Body Fat Solution

The program encourages slow and steady progress. You can expect results fast enough to keep you motivated, yet slow enough that you don't risk your health. Extreme weight-loss competitions and reality shows may be entertaining and even inspiring, but they're about as far from reality as you can get. If you're sincere about getting lean and staying lean, then this endeavor shouldn't be a race, but a journey of learning and gradual self-improvement.

Instant gratification and quick fixes are rejected in favor of lifestyle changes. Rapid and extreme weight-loss programs may be tempting but are unrealistic for most people and usually produce only short-term results. A true solution doesn't deceive you with temporary water-weight loss or the short-lived exhilaration of quick results that can't be maintained.

The Body Fat Solution is not a weight-loss program, it's a fat-burning program. Muscle is weight that you want to keep. Fat is the weight you want to shed. You will typically aim for a goal of about two pounds per week of body fat loss. If you have a lot of fat to lose, then losing up to 1 percent of your total body weight is a sensible weekly goal.

This program has no dogmatic exercise prescriptions, rigid food lists, or strict carbohydrate counts. As you read each chapter, you'll be amazed at the freedom you have in your exercise and food choices. If an exercise burns a lot of calories, you can do it, If a food contains lots of nutrients and relatively few calories, you can eat it. You can even choose how many carbohydrates you want to eat instead of being restricted to a predetermined limit. This sense of freedom makes the program easy to fit your lifestyle.

To succeed in the long run, you need strategies for controlling your appetite. On the Body Fat Solution nutrition plan, you'll experience less hunger than you would on other diets, because the calorie reduction is small; you get to eat something every three hours, and the foods you eat will make you feel fuller on fewer calories.

Many people are concerned that a fat-loss meal plan must be bland or unpalatable. Not true. You can eat delicious foods and still lose body fat. In fact, you can eat anything you want as long as you understand the key to enjoying your favorite foods appropriately. The answer is calorie control and moderation. Diets that force you to eat foods you dislike are usually among the first to fail, regardless of what other virtues they may possess. On this plan, there are no forbidden foods.

If you've struggled with excess body fat in the past, rest assured it's not because you had a "diet pill deficiency." The Body Fat Solution does not promote or require any pills, drinks, or supplements. You can take a multivitamin/mineral and other supplements if you choose, but they are not mandatory. So-called "fat burners" play no part in this program.

Food, not individual nutrients, is the focus of the Body Fat Solution, and whole, natural foods will be the secret to your success. You will eat common foods you can find readily at any grocery store or natural foods market in almost any country. If you ever get bored with your menu or can't find a particular food, substitutions are a cinch.

Even more exciting, you'll find this program is socially acceptable. You'll be able to eat at restaurants with friends, attend social functions, and enjoy holidays without worrying about your diet. When your friends see you eating chocolate, ice cream, or your other favorite foods, they'll be mystified at how you continue to get leaner. Even your meal schedule will be flexible. You can enjoy three traditional sit-down meals with snacks in between. Eating more frequent meals, as many athletes and bodybuilders do, is an option, not a requirement.

The Body Fat Solution is all about choice. It was engineered to fit your lifestyle, not disrupt it. Instead of being victim of a negative environment and peer pressure, you'll learn how to recruit your friends, family, peers, and coworkers as a part of your success team. You'll quickly discover that surrounding yourself with winners helps you become a winner yourself.

What You Must Give for the Body Fat Solution to Work for You

With this brief preview of what's in store, you're probably feeling more optimistic than ever about finally following through with your self-promises to get the body you've always wanted. However, it's important to balance your enthusiasm with reality; there's no such thing as something for nothing. The results you get will come in direct proportion to the effort you invest. There are many ways to increase efficiency, but there are no shortcuts.

In the beginning, you must use your willpower and personal discipline. There's no secret to getting started. You simply decide and then take your first step. With each subsequent step, the next one becomes easier and more habitual while your confidence builds and your momentum increases. Willpower gets you started, but only habit keeps you going.

To change your body you must reprogram your thinking and change your belief systems. *This is the key to developing positive habits.* Your unconscious mind is powerful beyond comprehension. If you've ever started a fitness plan with the best intentions but then sabotaged yourself, it's because you were using only your conscious mind while negative unconscious programming continued to run unchecked.

As you begin this journey, be prepared to accept responsibility for your results, for better or worse. You must adopt the Body Fat Solution winner's creed: *You can either make excuses or get results, but you can't do both.*

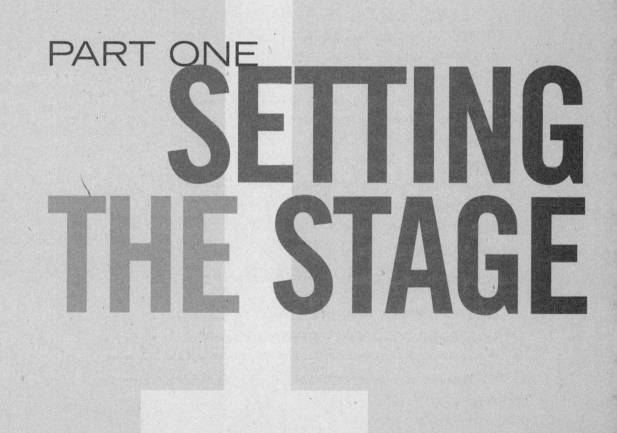

PART ONE

SETTING THE STAGE

Body Fat

CHAPTER ONE

A New **Understanding**
of the **Problem**

> **VERY** often when making a decision about something, we don't use all the relevant available information; we use, instead, only a single, highly representative piece of the total. And an isolated piece of information, even though it normally counsels us correctly, can lead us to clearly stupid mistakes.
>
> —ROBERT CIALDINI, PH.D., SOCIAL PSYCHOLOGIST

Imagine a roundtable conference of all the world's weight-loss experts debating the real reason for the body fat problem. The roster includes distinguished research scientists, exercise physiologists, medical doctors, personal trainers, dietitians, book authors, psychologists, pharmaceutical companies, supplement manufacturers, and any other authority or group with a connection to the weight-loss industry.

I imagine the debate going something like this:

3

Registered dietitian: "Low fat is the answer. Dietary fat has more calories, the lowest thermic effect, and it's most easily converted into fat. Research shows that high dietary fat intake correlates to high body fat."

Low-carb-diet book author #1: "Yes, but correlation doesn't equal causation. It's not the fat, it's the carbs. The current health advice to eat more breads, cereals, and grains is making us fat and killing us."

Balanced-diet book author: "Demonizing entire foods groups doesn't help anyone, it only confuses people. There are good carbs and bad carbs, good fats and bad fats. It's all about balancing the three macronutrients: protein, carbohydrates, and fats."

Low-carb-diet book author #2: "It's not just the carbs. When overweight people eat carbs, their blood sugar and insulin go out of control. The hormone insulin is the real cause of obesity."

Supplement-company research director: "High insulin can block fat burning and fat release, but that doesn't mean insulin causes obesity. Thyroid is the real issue. Fix your thyroid and you'll fix any body fat problem. By the way, we just released a new supplement that optimizes your thyroid gland."

Research scientist #1: "It's definitely hormones, but the hormone leptin controls everything, even the thyroid. Mark my words, leptin will be the 'next big thing' in fat loss.

Research scientist #2: "You make it sound as if we have control over our body chemistry. If people are born with the fat gene, it's going to be harder for them to lose weight and they have to accept that. Tell them to blame their parents."

Personal trainer: "Blaming it on genetics is a cop-out. We were genetically built to be active. Our ancestors did physical labor to survive or make a living. Exercise is the solution. Send any overweight person to our training studio and you'll see."

Bariatric surgeon: "But how is an obese person supposed to exercise? Not only that, overweight people have malfunctioning appetite regulation systems, so gastric bypass is the sure thing. Our practice performed over a thousand procedures last year."

Supplement-company sales rep: "Why would you cut someone open when we have natural appetite suppressants? Our researchers discovered an herb from the Amazon rain forest and it kills hunger like you wouldn't believe. We did ten million in sales last year. What does that tell you?"

Pharmaceutical-company spokesperson: "It tells us you have a great marketing department. Your intentions are good, but herbs are too weak. We believe obesity is a result of excess production of ZXX, the appetite-stimulating stomach hormone we just discovered. We've already got a breakthrough drug in clinical trials that will control this hormonal monster."

Natural-foods advocate: "People are eating too much, but it's not their fault. Blame it on supersizing and modern processed food. We don't need drugs, supplements, or surgery. We should sue the fast-food corporations and then we have to reeducate the public about natural foods and portion control."

Hypnotherapist: "You're all missing something. If someone can't stay motivated to do what has to be done, then even the best diet or workout is worthless. Behavior change is the key and it's all in the subconscious mind. That's why hypnosis is the only true solution."

If you think this fictitious scenario sounds too outrageous to be true, or if you found this dialogue humorous, then think again and don't laugh too hard. The debate you just heard is remarkably close to the real state of the weight-loss industry as we progress into the twenty-first century.

Who's *Really* Right? What's the *Real* Cause of Obesity?

You might be saying to yourself, "The real cause of body fat is obvious: we eat too much, we eat the wrong foods, and we don't exercise enough." If you did, you'd be right. Body fat is the result of a surplus of caloric energy, caused by a sedentary lifestyle and an environment encouraging excess caloric intake. If you stop there, however, you won't truly understand why there's an obesity epidemic today. You must dig deeper and ask more questions about root causes, questions like:

- Why is it so hard to balance calorie input with output?
- What prevents me from eating better and exercising more?
- Why is it tough to put into practice what I already know?
- What emotional and psychological factors are blocking me from succeeding?
- Is my physical or social environment sabotaging me?
- Could some of the information I've believed about exercise be wrong?
- Was the last diet I tried too complex to apply consistently with success?
- Was my last diet too extreme to stay on long enough to reach my goals?
- Was I able to reach my goal but unable to maintain it?

When you ask these types of questions, you start to realize that body fat isn't an isolated issue, but rather it's a bundle of physical, mental, emotional, and social problems producing a single physical symptom. Removing body fat is not simply a matter of going on a diet—it's a much more complex issue, involving every area of your life.

That's why I didn't write this book about an isolated nutrient, a single hormone, a lone diet technique, the latest exercise trend, or a novel discovery that might someday turn into a supplement or pharmaceutical. The Body Fat Solution is a total life program addressing all the root causes and approaching the problem from every angle.

The Body Fat Solution Three-Step Problem-Solving Formula

One of the more famous approaches to solving problems was created by American physicist Richard Feynman. He called it the "problem-solving algorithm" and it contained three ultrasimple steps:

1. understand the problem;
2. think very hard;
3. write out the answer.

Without a doubt, a solution always begins with understanding the problem, but when it comes to body fat, that's often easier said than done. Getting rid of body fat appears simple on paper, but proves more difficult in practice. To get to the bottom of it requires a new problem-solving approach specific to health and fitness, and that's exactly what I've created.

Like the Feynman formula, the Body Fat Solution problem-solving formula also has three rules:

1. **Understand cause and effect.** You can't solve a problem simply by treating the symptoms. We live in a universe governed by many natural laws. The granddaddy of all them all is the law of cause and effect, which says that every condition or effect can be traced back to one or more causes. A true solution must uncover and treat the cause, and if there's more than one cause, you must find and address all of them.

2. **Think differently.** The second rule, and we can thank Einstein for this one, is that *you can't solve a problem at the same level of thinking that created it*. Most people think constantly, but they think mostly about the same things they did yesterday. Usually, they're mulling over their problems and thinking about what they don't want, rather than focusing on solutions and thinking about what they do want. Thoughts are causes, while behaviors and conditions are effects. Therefore, if you keep thinking the same thoughts, you'll continue producing the same results. Thinking hard is not enough, you have to think differently.

3. **Act on the answer.** You must take action. One of the biggest reasons for failure is having a large gap between what you know and what you actually do. From the ancient Greek comes a word called *praxis*, which refers to the practice or doing of what you already know. Having a solution in mind

doesn't guarantee results. Success comes when you put knowledge and understanding into action.

The True Causes of Body Fat and the Problems That Perpetuate It

With this new approach to problem solving, your first step is to understand some of the deeper causes and the real problems that could be preventing you from getting leaner. Many of these may not be what you expect.

PROBLEM: Information Isolation

If you've searched for weight-loss advice on the Internet in the past few years, then you're probably familiar with information overload. A lesser-known off-shoot is what I call information isolation. This is the attempt to treat body fat with a single, isolated strategy that doesn't acknowledge the whole gamut of causes.

Your body is made up of many diverse and dynamic systems. Your mind is even more complex than you can fathom. These mental and physical sides of you are intertwined, and together they create the behavior and physiology that result in weight loss, gain, or maintenance.

Pulling out one piece of a complex process and calling it the Holy Grail is the norm in the weight-loss marketplace, but it's an approach destined to fail. For example, if an entire program revolves around one nutrient such as a vitamin, mineral, or macronutrient or a single hormone such as cortisol, insulin, or leptin, it should be viewed as incomplete at best. If one hormone or nutrient is presented as the single cause or the be-all and end-all solution, watch out. It never is.

SOLUTION: Synergy

Synergy is when two or more separate ingredients act together to create a whole that's greater than the sum of its parts. Two pieces of wood fastened together can hold more weight than the total held by each separately. Human synergy is where people "mastermind," join forces, and the ideas and achievements they produce together exceed what they could produce individually. Synergy in health and fitness means putting all the individual components together into a lifestyle. The Body Fat Solution is not nutrition, exercise, mind-set, emotions, or social support, it's all these things working together.

You may have seen the effects of one weight-loss strategy in isolation before, but it pales in comparison to the results you'll get when you put multiple strategies together. When you diet, you may lose weight, but if you add aerobic exercise, you get better results than with diet alone. If you combine the diet and aerobics with strength training, again your results multiply. When you add mental, emotional, and social support strategies to your diet and exercise program, results multiply exponentially because you've added the tools for compliance and long-term maintenance.

PROBLEM: Dogmatic Beliefs

One of the biggest reasons that information isolation persists is because of dogmatic beliefs. The dogmatic authority gets so emotionally attached or financially vested in his theories and methods, he'd rather die than admit he was wrong. Theories are proposed in a way that they can't be tested, critical analysis is opposed, debate is avoided, and science is rejected or selectively quoted. His motto: "It's my way or the highway."

Beliefs are like treasured possessions, so most people don't like to part with them. But unlike many authorities, the real scientist discards old hypotheses when they're proven incorrect and then spins new ones, a continuous process of discovery that expands knowledge and brings all of us closer to the truth.

SOLUTION: Choice and Flexibility

Cybernetics is the study of systems control, as in computer science, artificial intelligence, or human psychology, where feedback from output is used to modify subsequent input. In the field of cybernetics, there's a concept that's extremely useful in your endeavors to reduce body fat. It's called the "law of requisite variety." This law says that in any system, human or mechanical, if all else is equal, the more flexibility and variety you have in your choices, the more power you have to control your results.

Applying this law requires that you put yourself into a feedback loop where you execute a course of action and then measure your progress at frequent intervals. It also requires paying close attention to your results to determine whether your current plan is working. Based on your results, you can continue forward with the same plan or make adjustments.

Repeating more of the same actions can only produce more of the same results. If your plan isn't working, you need to change your plan and then get back into action. If you lack options or you're bound by dogmatic rules, then you're stuck. That's why the Body Fat Solution is focused on increasing your choices rather than taking them away.

PROBLEM: Baloney

A huge part of the body fat problem is the fads, frauds, fakes, and downright weird stuff sold in the marketplace today. Collectively, we'll call this "baloney," and it includes all the products and programs that have no scientific evidence supporting their claims. Baloney creates a problem because it adds to the information overload. It could also be costing you a fortune. Millions of men and women get scammed every year, heading down the wrong path. Their sense of frustration builds with each failed attempt.

If there's no science behind it, then how do weight-loss companies keep getting away with selling baloney and why do people keep buying it? The Federal Trade Commission (FTC) in the United States and watchdog organizations in other countries do their best to monitor and prosecute fraud, but it's so rampant they can't even put a dent in it. Most people don't investigate before they invest—they buy on impulse or emotion and advertisers know how to hit your emotional hot buttons. And where there's demand, there will always be supply.

SOLUTION: Baloney Detector

The best defense against baloney is a good baloney detector. In his brilliant book on the virtues of science, *The Demon-Haunted World*, Carl Sagan devoted an entire chapter to the art of "baloney detection." It's a set of skills you have to learn and hone, which includes understanding the scientific method, developing critical-thinking skills, and viewing claims with a skeptical eye.

Key skills of baloney detection include:

- getting independent confirmation of the facts;
- encouraging and participating in constructive debate;
- considering science as the only authority;
- creating more than one hypothesis;
- avoiding attachment to your own ideas;
- being sure that claims and results can be measured;
- making certain that claims can be tested;
- realizing that the simplest explanation is usually the correct one.

I'm not suggesting you should become a closed-minded skeptic, only that you should develop the skills to think critically and evaluate claims scientifically. If it sounds too good to be true, assume it is until proven otherwise. Remember one last thing: some baloney actually works, but it's all in the mind—the placebo effect is very real.

PROBLEM: The Extreme Approach

Unlike baloney, extreme approaches can actually produce results, sometimes very quickly. The problem is, most people never stick with them long enough to reach their long-term goal or they suffer and deprive themselves to get there.

There are hundreds of ways to lose weight with extreme diet and exercise regimes. But what happens next? If you pursue extreme dieting with teeth-grinding willpower, you'll probably have a hard time maintaining your lighter weight because extreme diets set your body up for weight regain. According to most obesity researchers, at least 90 percent of dieters will gain back all the weight they lost. Many even experience a rebound effect, ending up with more body fat than they had in the first place.

SOLUTION: The Moderate Approach

"Extreme transformations" have been glorified in television and advertising to such a degree that anything but a dramatic makeover today is sneered at. When it comes to body fat, extreme approaches often produce the most impressive results in the short term, but they almost never work over the long term. The solution is the moderate approach.

Moderation might seem like compromise but not in the case of weight control. In *The 7 Habits of Highly Effective People*, Steven Covey points out that in a synergistic situation, taking the middle ground is not a compromise, it means "higher" as in the apex of a pyramid. From a long-term perspective, this simply means a maintainable lifestyle.

An effective fat-burning program doesn't have to be a radical departure from your usual year-round eating habits. To burn fat, you must consistently eat fewer calories than you burn, but even your calorie reduction should be moderate, not extreme. In long-term body fat control, slow and steady wins it almost every time.

PROBLEM: Complexity

If you have an analytical or inquiring mind, then my guess is that you're not satisfied with being told that something works. You probably have an insatiable curiosity to find out all the details about how and why it works. However, it's not more details and explanations of mechanisms that will make you more successful. In fact, the opposite may be true. When you're given too many choices or if there's too much detail in a process, it's common to make no decisions or postpone action while you continue analyzing and researching.

Body fat is the most complex, yet the simplest problem known to humanity. At its most basic level, it's nothing but a matter of energy balance. "Eat fewer calories than you burn" is the correct advice, but not as easy as it sounds. The complexity problem comes into play because energy balance is dynamic. Dozens, and maybe even hundreds, of factors can shift your body's energy balance equation and affect whether calories are "partitioned" into or out of your body's fat stores or lean tissues.

SOLUTION: Simplicity

In the fourteenth century, English philosopher William of Occam proposed that "entities should not be multiplied unnecessarily." This decision-making principle, which became known as Occam's razor, means that the simplest solution is usually the correct one. Other great minds agreed. Over twenty-four hundred years ago, Socrates said that the best solution to any problem was probably the one with the fewest number of steps. Einstein said to make everything as simple as possible, but not any simpler.

You might think that the program with the most information, the most steps, and the most attention to detail will be the most effective one. That might be true if you actually applied all those details, but in practice, it's the complex process reduced to the fewest number of steps, without losing the essentials, that produces the best results. Simplification doesn't imply that details are unimportant, only that you must first put the essentials in place before thinking about the details.

PROBLEM: Noncompliance

Contrary to popular opinion, diets do work. Any diet that puts you in a consistent caloric deficit can produce weight loss. The problem is, most of them don't work for long. The real issue is compliance. Many diets are too extreme to follow long term, and most people lack the motivation to stick with any low-calorie diet long enough to get good results.

In 2005, a study was published in the *Journal of the American Medical Association* comparing four of the most popular diet programs with approaches that include carbohydrate restriction, fat restriction, calorie restriction, and macronutrient balance. The researchers made some surprising observations.

First, they said that each diet worked. All four modestly reduced body weight. Second, they noted that the amount of weight lost was related to how well the subjects could follow the diet. They discovered that any of the four diets could reduce body weight, but only for those who could actually stick with them, which was the minority. Third, they found the diets on the extremes—very low fat and very low carb—had the lowest compliance rates.

They concluded that none of the diets produced satisfactory adherence and that compliance decreased at a similar rate over time for all four of the programs. The researcher's final comment pointed the way toward the solution: "To manage a national epidemic of excess body weight, practical techniques to increase dietary adherence rates are urgently needed."

SOLUTION: Adherence Tools and Compliance Rules

It's only natural for each of the various diet programs to claim that its approach is the best. Most of us would also agree that certain diets are clearly more effective than others in terms of greater fat loss, better muscle retention, and improved health. However, the best program in the truest sense is not the most effective program, but rather an effective program you can actually stick with long term.

The harsh reality is that not sticking with it may be the biggest problem of all. This teaches us that we can't look only to the fields of nutrition and exercise science for solutions; we also must look to the field of psychology. Some of the best tools for increased sustainability and compliance are mental, emotional, and even social.

These compliance tools are sometimes as simple as shifts in your thoughts, beliefs, and attitudes, which you'll learn about in the upcoming chapters.

When you use these tools and rules diligently, they can help you more consistently follow the Body Fat Solution principles or any other nutrition and exercise program you choose.

PROBLEM: Prioritizing What's New

If you're like most people, you get bored quickly. That's not necessarily a bad thing, it's simply human nature. You demand new reading, new recreation, new cars, new possessions, and new entertainment. If the newspaper said the same thing every day, would you keep reading it? If your favorite TV show kept running the same episode, would you keep watching it? Probably not, and it's the same with diet programs.

The difference is, while your mind and ego require fresh stimulation, your body requires a small number of essentials every day. Your success with losing body fat will come from repeating a small handful of fundamentals over and over again. It's kind of boring, but necessary. If that's true, then why is there a new diet, a new pill, or a new exercise gadget released every month or an authority claiming that a scientific breakthrough has revolutionized weight loss?

The answer is simple: having a new hook is necessary for commercial success. Companies that fail to innovate or release new models go out of business. The media is under constant pressure to seek out new stories and angles. The marketplace will always demand "the next big thing in weight loss" for as long as human beings continue to get bored and want what's new rather than what's important.

Staying informed and up to date is virtuous. However, appeal to novelty is a logical fallacy. Just because it's new doesn't mean it is better. If you abandon ship and hop from one trend to the next, always looking for the next big thing, you risk losing sight of the fundamentals or second-guessing yourself even when your current approach is already working.

SOLUTION: Prioritizing Fundamentals

What's most important is focusing on the essentials and repeating the fundamentals day after day. A classic example comes from professional football. When Vince Lombardi took over the Green Bay Packers the year after they suffered their worst season ever, everyone asked him what he was going to do to turn the team around: "Are you going to change the playbooks? Are you going to change the players? What are you going to do differently?" He replied, "I'm not going to change anything, we're just going to get brilliant on the basics."

How basic, you ask? At the beginning of the season, Lombardi gave a speech to his entire team, rookies and veterans alike. He began by holding out a familiar-looking prolate spheroid and saying, "We're going back to fundamentals. Gentlemen, this is a football." Lombardi believed that fundamentals were the answer, and he became one of the winningest coaches in NFL history.

It's the same with winning at weight control. You must get brilliant on the basics. You probably already know most of the fundamentals intuitively. If you haven't mastered them, then nothing new that comes down the pike will be of much use to you. Without question, there will be important new discoveries made, but there's no such thing as a "new fundamental."

PROBLEM: Quick-fix Disease

Brian Tracy, one of the world's foremost experts on success psychology, once said that there are two "diseases" running rampant across America and much of the industrialized world today. They're not physical diseases, they're diseases of mind, emotions, and character, which hold millions of people back from achieving their long-term goals.

One of them is called quick-fix disease. People with this affliction want to take a pill, go to sleep, and wake up skinny. They're suckers for the latest fat-burning cream or steroid-replacement scam. They impulsively buy "miracle" solutions that they haven't researched and know nothing about. They search for instant cures to solve health problems that may have taken a lifetime to develop. They look for overnight shortcuts to fitness goals that normally take months or even years to attain. Saddest and most ironic, they often waste years of their lives on this fruitless quest, with no results to show for it.

This isn't the same as wanting to find more efficient ways of reaching your goals. There's a principle in psychology called the law of least effort which says that no intelligent human being will choose a slower way to achieve a goal when a faster way is available. In contrast, quick-fix disease is contracted when people want a way to reach their goals faster than nature intended.

SOLUTION: Long-term Perspective

Long-term perspective includes setting long-term goals, but also much more. Goals are essential and you'll learn more about them in Chapter Five, but each goal is only a stepping-stone, not an end point. Without a bigger vision and purpose for each area of your life, you won't have the motivational drive that keeps you going and you'll be more likely to fall for quick fixes.

Long-term perspective also means that you consider the ultimate consequences of all your behaviors and decisions. Before you act, you must project yourself into the future. What would be the long-term consequences of going on a radical diet, an extreme training program, or a risky drug? The more you think about long-term consequences at the moment of every decision, the better your decisions will be.

Making decisions with the long term in mind often implies sacrifice. Like moderation, "sacrifice" is a misunderstood word. Many people think sacrifice means deprivation or giving something up. What sacrifice really means is giving up something of a lower nature in the present to receive something of a higher nature in the future.

It's easy for a twenty-year-old to live only for today and shrug off the long-term consequences. It may seem ridiculous to set twenty-five-year goals, but consider this: I've never met a forty-five-year-old who didn't care about his health and appearance, but I've met many who regretted not caring twenty-five years ago.

PROBLEM: Something-for-Nothing Disease

Just as you'd take a faster way to achieve a goal rather than a slower way, it's also normal to want the easier way rather than the harder way. This is neither good nor bad, nor is it necessarily laziness; again, it's just human nature. The difference is, an efficient person is willing to do the hard work but simply wants to do it in the most economical manner possible. The person with something-for-nothing disease wants a result or reward without doing the work at all.

People with something-for-nothing disease want weight loss without dieting, fitness without exercise, and health while eating, drinking, and smoking whatever they want. As they pursue methods that promise results without work, their health and body composition fail to improve. Sometimes it gets worse because many of the quick fixes, such as drugs, surgery, or starvation, come with serious physical side effects.

Thomas Jefferson once said, "The worst day of a man's life is when he sits down and begins thinking about how he can get something for nothing." Something-for-nothing disease is like a virus that easily spreads from one area of your life to another and gradually chips away at your character, erodes your self-discipline, and diminishes your self-esteem.

SOLUTION: Hard and Efficient Work

I highly recommend reading Ralph Waldo Emerson's nineteen-page essay on compensation (it's in the public domain and freely available online). Although it's written in somewhat stoic and metaphysical nineteenth-century prose, if you can plod your way through it and extract the central message, your life will never be the same again. The law of compensation is not only a powerful principle of economics, but also a universal law that governs every aspect of your life, your body, and your health.

You can only receive in direct proportion to what you give. There's perfect equity and balance in the universe. "Tit for tat, measure for measure, give and it shall be given," said Emerson. "Nothing ventured, nothing gained. Thou shalt be paid exactly for what thou hast done, no more, no less. Who doth not work shall not eat. No offense goes unchastised. Honest service cannot come to loss. Every virtue is rewarded. Every stroke shall be repaid. What will you have, quoth God; pay for it and take it."

It has often been said that you don't need to work hard, only smarter. That's incorrect. Success requires hard work as well as smart work. There are always more efficient ways of doing things and it's wise to pursue them, but there's no way around hard work. As for goods and services, you must pay a fair price for everything else in life.

Setting a worthy goal for something you want, then pursuing and reaching it through determination, discipline, and hard work changes the very fiber of your being. You become a stronger person, not just physically, but also mentally and emotionally. Work develops your character, strengthens your discipline, and boosts your self-esteem.

PROBLEM: It's-Not-My-Fault Disease

I've identified a third "disease" of the mind and emotions, called it's-not-my-fault. People with this ailment tend to cast blame, make excuses, and absolve themselves of responsibility for all their negative results and failures. Blame is always placed squarely on someone or something outside themselves. They use excuses to defend their limiting beliefs, to justify their lack of action, to explain why they believe something can't be done, or to let themselves off the hook of personal accountability.

It takes self-discipline and self-mastery to overcome this tendency. If you're not careful, blaming and excuse-making can become a habitual knee-jerk reaction every time you're confronted with an obstacle or challenge. If you indulge in it's-not-my-fault disease, you're giving up control of your life and playing the victim. Chronic blamers and excuse-makers rarely improve and never reach a high level of success because if they believe they're not in control of their results, then how can they change them?

SOLUTION: Accepting Responsibility

The cure for it's-not-my-fault disease is responsibility. If you have a lean, fit body, it wasn't luck. It wasn't an accident. You did it. You deserve the credit. If you have an overweight, unfit body, it didn't happen by chance. It was not an accident. You did it. You deserve the blame. You can't have it only one way.

I'm not saying you should dismiss the conditions outside of your control that might make weight loss more challenging. Genetics play a role in body fat, and some diseases and prescription drugs can also make fat loss more difficult. However, many people confuse "difficult" with "impossible." Another definition of responsibility is "response-ability," which means free will—your ability to choose your response to any situation. The question isn't whether difficulties exist that make losing weight harder, but rather how you respond to them.

Three of the most powerful words in the English language are "I am responsible." It's tough to do, but when the day comes that you can say those words, believe them, and mean them, it will be one of the most liberating moments of your life. Taking responsibility for all your results, for better or for worse, is taking back your power to create results in your life.

PROBLEM: Negative Environment and Social Pressure

There's an old fisherman's story that if you put a crab in a bucket, you have to put a lid on the bucket, otherwise the crab will climb out. However, if you put a bunch of crabs in a bucket, you don't need to put a lid on it because if one crab tries to escape, the other crabs will pull it back down.

Unfortunately, a lot of people are like crabs. Anytime you announce you want to achieve a big goal, these people will line up to tell you why you can't do it, as the biographies of all the world's greatest inventors will show you. If you begin anyway, they'll be there again to tell you you're wasting your time. If you start to move forward and become successful while the others do not, the ones "left behind" will often feel jealousy, resentment, or contempt for you. If they can't succeed themselves, they won't want you to succeed either, so they'll try to drag you down, like crabs in a bucket.

Almost everywhere around you, negative forces are trying to pull you down. Regrettably, the people closest to you can sometimes be the biggest negative influences of all. A large part of socializing involves eating and drinking together and the nature of those habits can easily rub off on you. Poor choices are easier to justify when others around you are making those same poor choices.

As you're beginning to control your portion sizes and eat healthier foods, you may hear sarcastic or hostile comments like, "How can you live on that rabbit food? Don't you want more? Don't you miss real food?" Once you begin getting in good shape, others say, "Isn't that enough? If you lose any more weight you'll be anorexic. How do you live like that? Life is too short to be in the gym all the time. Live a little."

SOLUTION: Positive Environment and Social Support

Experts on social influence say that your financial income will usually equal the average of your five closest friends. I think that's pretty darn accurate. I also believe that your health is your greatest wealth, and the condition of your body will be about equal to the average of your five closest friends. The good news about social influence is that it works in both directions. That's why you must guard yourself against negative people, environments, and influences and build your social network into a fortress of positivity.

Your mental and emotional energy is too precious to squander on negative, pessimistic people. Your interactions with others should leave you energized and charged up, not depressed and depleted. Emotional vampires will suck you dry if you let them. You must do everything in your power to protect your positive energy and keep negative people away from you.

You can't choose your family, but you can petition their support and recruit your current circle of friends to join you in your new fitness and lifestyle changes. At the same time, you can always make new friends, join groups of like-minded positive people, hire coaches or trainers, find mentors and role models, and put yourself in a more positive environment in your free time when you're not at home or at work.

Summing Up the Problems

Were you at all surprised by this list of problems? Maybe you were expecting the list to present issues like insulin resistance, hormonal imbalance, genetics, appetite regulation, supersized portions, sedentary lifestyles, and moving away from our evolutionary diet. I easily could have focused on those topics and in fact I will mention some of them throughout the rest of this book.

Instead, you heard about problems with solutions such as responsibility, synergy, flexibility, moderation, critical thinking, getting back to basics, and hard work. Why? First, because I always teach mental dynamics before physical strategies. Second, because regardless of whether you follow the exercise and nutrition programs suggested in part two of this book, or you choose some other nutrition and exercise philosophy, these mental and emotional solutions still apply to you.

Unless you understand root causes and the true nature of the problem, and unless you prepare your mind for success by eliminating potential mental and emotional blocks up front, when you do get to the physical side of this process, you're likely to find yourself getting in your own way and sabotaging your own success. Erroneous thinking, negative attitudes, limiting beliefs, and destructive emotions can all block you from succeeding even if you have the best nutrition and training program in the world.

In the rest of part one, you'll learn more about the importance of your attitudes, thoughts, and beliefs and how the right ones set the stage for your long-term success. Thinking critically and taking a long, hard look at what you believe is the first step. With deep and honest analysis, it's often shocking to see how many of our most cherished beliefs actually turn out to be myths.

Body Fat Myths and Why We Believe Them

IF we don't practice the tough habits of thought, we cannot hope to solve the truly serious problems that face us, and we risk becoming a nation of suckers, a world of suckers, up for grabs by the next charlatan who saunters along.

—CARL SAGAN, ASTRONOMER

Some people believe in really weird stuff about diet and exercise. In fact, millions of people believe myths and fallacies about body fat and weight loss. Maybe you're not one of them, but then again, intelligent and clearheaded people are as susceptible as anyone. Michael Shermer, a skeptic and columnist for *Scientific American*, put it well when he said, "Smart people believe weird things because they are skilled at defending beliefs they arrived at for non-smart reasons."

23

With so much information overload today, it takes more than intelligence to see through myths and misconceptions. If you want to avoid being a victim of fitness fraud and diet deception and start getting better results, then you must develop and practice new habits of thought. These include critical thinking and healthy skepticism.

Some people argue, "What harm does it do to believe in something even if it turns out to be untrue?" I speak from experience when I say that health and fitness myths are far from harmless. They cost you wasted time and usually money, many can hold back your progress, and some can be extremely damaging to your body and your health.

Failure to think critically and scientifically has led to great tragedies in human history, including epidemics. Today we're suffering from an epidemic of obesity and all the related health problems, including type 2 diabetes, cardiovascular disease, hypertension, and metabolic syndrome. Excess body fat isn't simply a frustrating cosmetic problem, it's a quality-of-life problem. Myths about body fat and weight loss only perpetuate it.

Question Everything

There are many areas in life where careful analysis of claims is important. In the fitness and weight-loss marketplace, it's imperative. Some people argue that skepticism is nothing but cynicism and refusal to accept new ideas. I agree that some skeptics may come across as closed-minded curmudgeons, but I believe that true critical and scientific thinking is quite the opposite.

A critical thinker doesn't necessarily approach every claim or belief with a presupposition that it's false or with the implicit objective of debunking it. In the highest form of critical thinking, a claim, belief, or hypothesis is examined from a neutral point of view, with no bias either way.

Since we see the world through our own perceptual filters, it's not easy to analyze a new idea with an open mind and a neutral viewpoint. Scrutinizing our own long-held beliefs can be one of the most difficult challenges we'll ever face. Critical thinking begins with accepting the possibility that some of our most cherished beliefs could be wrong. It can be humbling or painful to accept this, but if we fail to be discerning and critical, we risk becoming vulnerable to the charlatans who intend to bamboozle us with their baloney. You must question new claims and challenge old beliefs. How do you know what you believe is true? How do you know what isn't so?

Eight Reasons We Are Susceptible to Weight-Loss Myths

Before taking a close look at each of the major body fat myths, it's important to examine how you arrived at your beliefs about health, fitness, and weight loss. If you can't identify the source, then you're in danger of slipping into old patterns of thinking and falling for the same old myths each time they reappear in new clothes.

REASON #1: Social Proof, Conformity, and Appeal to the Masses

Usually you assume a behavior is appropriate if a lot of other people are doing it. This is known as social proof. Psychologists tell us this phenomenon also applies to beliefs. We believe what we do because it's what most other people believe. In general, this appears to be reasonable. It does, however, have a huge downside. What if everyone else is wrong? What if those people are also looking at what other people are doing? The result is "pluralistic ignorance," where we have followers following the followers and few people thinking for themselves.

In *The Strangest Secret*, the classic gold recording on personal achievement in America, Earl Nightingale said that only 3 percent of people are successful. He suggested that the reason for the low success rate was conformity. But the real trouble was that they were following the wrong people—the 97 percent who don't succeed. Continuing this line of reasoning, Nightingale proposed that if we look at what the majority does and do the exact opposite, the chances are, we'll be on the track toward success.

REASON #2: Appeal to Authority and Loyalty to Gurus

It seems only natural to depend on information from the "experts." Their opinions are believable because they're based on credentials, reputation, and experience.

Sometimes you even grant "fitness expert" status on the basis of physique alone. Personally, I give a higher level of respect to anyone who walks the walk and displays excellent fitness and physique. You should, however, keep in mind that some of the worst advice in our field has been given by people with some of the best bodies, and experts are not always correct.

Being an expert in one area also doesn't imply expertise in another. Even brilliant medical doctors are often uninformed on the finer details of training and nutrition for weight loss, but when we see "M.D." after a name, we easily assume every word they speak about diet and exercise is accurate. Being a movie or TV personality is no indication of expertise outside the acting and broadcast journalism fields, yet most people put blind faith in celebrity endorsements on a regular basis. Celebrities are not experts. Many of them are famous only for being famous.

Even if someone is a genuine expert, he or she can be biased for numerous reasons, including political agenda, religious doctrine, personal ideology, professional ambition, or loyalty to a cause. Experts can also be biased by financial gain, as Carl Sagan explained:

PAID PRODUCT ENDORSEMENTS, especially by real or purported experts, constitute a steady rainfall of deception. They betray contempt for the intelligence of their customers. Today there are even commercials in which real scientists, some of considerable distinction, shill for corporations. They teach us that scientists too will lie for money.

The bottom line, and a basic premise of critical thinking, is that authorities don't matter, the facts do. All information must be analyzed critically and never accepted blindly. If the advice comes from people you respect and admire, then listen, but still verify.

REASON #3: Anecdotal Evidence and Testimonials

The vast majority of weight-loss products today attempt to prove their claims by using various forms of anecdotal evidence. In contrast to scientific evidence, anecdotes don't prove anything in a factual sense. Anecdotal evidence is usually little more than hearsay. For example, a friend of yours might say, "I know a guy who took this herb from the Amazon rain forest and lost sixty pounds." It's always prudent to question secondhand information. Get confirmation of the facts by finding the original source or at least people you trust who have firsthand knowledge of the facts.

Anecdotal evidence in the form of endorsements or testimonials is used in almost every advertisement because it's such a powerful persuasion tool. However, testimonials don't prove the products advertised were responsible for the claimed results, that the results were typical, or that the results happened at all.

The Federal Trade Commission and state attorney general's offices have been exposing more and more "miraculous" before-and-after photos for what they really are: setups and outright fakes. In January 2007, four well-known diet pill companies were sued by the FTC and ordered to pay $25 million in fines for false advertising and no evidence to back up their claims.

In one highly publicized case, a Los Angeles bodybuilder swore under oath that he was paid to stop working out and eat ice cream and doughnuts to fatten him up three weeks in advance of his "before" photo shoot. Then he used his bodybuilding expertise to get back in his usual top shape for the "after" photos.

According to an ABC 20/20 exposé about a similar case, a professional fitness model claimed in advertisements that she lost thirty-five pounds with the help of a popular fat-burner pill. However, the state attorney general discovered she had been pregnant and the "before" photo was taken shortly after she gave birth.

When stacked on top of scientific evidence, testimonials might add weight to an argument and give a balanced picture of what the real world says, compared to what science says. However, never accept testimonials at face value.

REASON #4: The News Said So

I'm sure most journalists are honest and they want to give you the facts accurately, objectively, and completely. You can't, however, always count on reporters to convey the facts correctly. Many of them may have no idea how to obtain independent verification of the facts through peer-reviewed studies. Some could be scientifically illiterate or unable to interpret research results.

Journalists are under great pressure to deliver the news while it's still new, and if possible, be the first to break a story. The success of the media also depends on delivering sensational news. An axiom among newscasters is, "If it bleeds, it leads." Dramatic stories are a must because fearmongering is big business; it sells newspapers, moves magazines off the newsstands, and raises ratings.

If you want to know who died, what hurricane is coming, or what burned down today, tune in to the news, because the media does a great job at reporting current events, especially negative ones. If you want to know how to solve a body fat or health problem, then take the news with a grain of salt. Your reporter may have rushed secondhand information to you without checking primary sources.

REASON #5: Confusing Correlation and Causation

Research has shown that spending a large amount of time watching television correlates to weight gain. Does this mean that the TV set causes you to get fat? Does the TV screen emit some kind of "fat radiation waves" that disrupt your cellular physiology and make you an adipose-storing machine? That conclusion is so far-fetched, it's silly to even consider. Yet people believe in far weirder things about diet and weight loss based purely on correlation.

The explanation for the link between TV watching and weight gain is simple: as a group, TV watchers tend to be inactive people and they're likely to habitually eat in front of the TV or engage in other unhealthy lifestyle behaviors.

Correlation does not equal causation. Confusing the two is one of the biggest sources of diet and weight-loss myths. Studying correlations provides valuable insights, but we have to be very careful not to jump prematurely to cause-and-effect conclusions.

There's also a correlation between eating in restaurants and weight gain. But does eating in restaurants *cause* weight gain? Again, the answer is no. Lots of people eat in restaurants, some quite often, and they stay perfectly fit and lean. What this correlation suggests is that as a group, people who eat frequently in restaurants are more likely to make poor choices and eat too much because restaurant meals typically contain more calorie-dense foods and serve more food than most people need. Being exposed to all kinds of appetizers, beverages, delicacies, and desserts on the menu also provides plenty of temptation.

Numerous studies have found a correlation between nighttime eating and weight gain. Does this mean that if you eat at night, the food will automatically turn into fat? Once again the answer is no. People who eat more at night tend to eat mindlessly in front of the TV, eat calorie-dense comfort foods, lose track of calories, or eat at night after already having fulfilled their energy needs during the day.

A final example is diet soda. How many times have you seen the headline "Diet Soda Makes You Fat"? This erroneous conclusion was based on studies that showed overweight people drank a lot of diet soda. But this doesn't mean the diet soda made them overweight. Even if diet soda triggered appetite, which is still uncertain, would that mean diet soda caused weight gain, or would weight gain be the result of the additional food eaten?

REASON #6: Confirmation Bias

To avoid information overload, our unconscious minds do a superb job at automatically deleting and distorting information based on our past prejudices and preferences. This is known as confirmation bias and there are two primary ways we do this. First, we seek only information that confirms our beliefs. Second, we resist or reject evidence that contradicts our beliefs.

We do this because it's psychologically comforting. It feels good to be right. It feels bad or embarrassing to be wrong. Even the most devoted scientists have to be careful to treat evidence from both sides evenhandedly because it's easy to allow commitment to a favorite theory or hypothesis to influence judgment. If continued, this type of selective thinking ultimately leads to closed-mindedness, poor decisions, discrimination, and justification for odd behaviors.

Your beliefs also influence how much information you seek. If the first evidence you find supports your viewpoints, you usually stop your search, having satisfied your need to confirm your point of view. However, if the first evidence you find contradicts your beliefs, then you tend to keep digging to try and uncover some evidence that supports your beliefs, or even proves that the first evidence you found was incorrect.

Shrewd marketers are well aware of these tendencies in human nature and use them to their advantage in peddling all kinds of baloney. For example, on many topics related to health and weight loss, the research is mixed and data in the scientific literature supports both sides. Advertisers often "cherry-pick" from mixed research, highlighting only the information that confirms their claims, while "forgetting" to mention the research that contradicts it.

REASON #7: Habitual Thinking and Appeal to Tradition

You probably have many eating and lifestyle habits that aren't working for you, but you repeat them every day without asking yourself why. If you've been training consistently, you may be working out a certain way because years ago someone told you that was the right way to do it. You've done it that way ever since. That's the power of habit.

I'll never forget how this happened to Brandon, one of my personal coaching protégés. When he started my program, he said his body fat had been stuck at 16 percent for the last six months, even though he was on the treadmill forty-five to sixty minutes nearly every day. He was utterly perplexed. He didn't see how it was physiologically possible to lift weights three times a week and do four to five hours of cardio per week without losing fat.

First I told him, "You could exercise ten hours a week and still be in energy balance. If your calorie intake matched your calorie output over the last six months, that's why you didn't lose weight." When I asked him how many calories he was burning and whether he'd increased the intensity of his workouts, a puzzled look came across his face. He said, "I thought I had to train longer and keep the intensity lower so I would burn fat and not sugar."

As it turned out, Brandon had fallen for the "fat-burning zone" myth, which actually tells you to intentionally slow down in order to burn more fat as fuel. This myth is based on a thread of scientific truth, but if you look at the big picture, you'll realize it's not even logical. To lose more weight, wouldn't you want to burn *more* calories, not fewer? If so, why would you slow down and burn fewer calories on purpose? Rather than worrying about what fuel he was burning during the workout, he should have focused on burning enough calories to maintain a twenty-four-hour calorie deficit every day.

All we had to do was increase his calorie burning while keeping a tight watch on his nutrition compliance. Twice a week he did a very intense twenty-five-minute interval workout and the other four days he stayed with the longer sessions, but he increased the intensity so he was burning more calories in the same time span. We actually *decreased* his training time and his body fat started dropping immediately.

Afterward, he told me he felt like kicking himself and that he'd wasted six months by repeating the same mistake over and over again. (He got over it, though, when he cracked the single digits ten weeks later and his body fat measurement hit 9.9 percent.)

The lesson is: if you do what you've always done, you'll get what you've always got. If you want a different result, do something different. Or as the humorous Demotivators calendar says: "Tradition . . . Just because you've always done it that way doesn't mean it's not incredibly stupid."

REASON #8: Wishful Thinking

It's tempting to form beliefs according to what we wish were true rather than on evidence or logic. It's more reassuring to believe that excess fat is not your fault and that a slow metabolism is to blame. It's more reassuring to believe that a health problem has nothing to do with the lifetime of habits that preceded it and it's entirely a matter of genetics. It's more reassuring to believe that eventually a weight-loss pill will be developed that gives you a fit and slim body without work. But wishing doesn't make any of these things so.

One concept that has become very popular in the personal success movement is the "law of attraction." This self-help principle suggests that if you focus your thoughts on and emotionalize a particular goal, while remaining open and expectant to receive it, then you will get it. As simplistic and New Age as it sounds, this is very consistent with how the unconscious mind works and with scientific principles of psychology. Many people, however, seem to have missed a step.

Positive thinking, affirmations, visualization, and other forms of mental training are effective ways to reprogram your unconscious mind. But the step that links thoughts and results is action. The main objective of all these mind techniques is to stimulate action and improve your physical performance. Sitting around thinking about what you want and daydreaming about what it would feel like to have it doesn't attract anything to you but dust and cobwebs.

The tendency to indulge in any kind of wishful thinking will only lead you down a path toward inaction, bad decisions, and poor results. It can also make you a target for marketers who dangle the promise of hope and tell you exactly what you want to hear.

The Eight Biggest Body Fat Myths

It's usually quite a wake-up call when you realize where you got your beliefs. Whether you were surprised, angered, enlightened, or all of the above, learning why you believe what you believe was an important and necessary first step. You're now better equipped to think critically and see things more clearly in the confusing nutrition and weight-loss marketplace. You'll also find it easier to recognize a myth when you hear one—and there are lots of them.

Hundreds of fitness and nutrition myths have been circulated through the gyms, social networks, and the popular media over the years, but eight myths in particular are responsible for more confusion, more misunderstanding, and more frustration to weight-loss seekers than all the others combined. If you buy into any of these myths, it can be the single obstacle that holds you back from better health and a leaner body.

MYTH #1: You can eat as much as you want and still lose weight

The cause of excess body fat is a positive energy balance, meaning you take in more energy (calories) than you burn. This is not a theory, as some diet authorities assert. It's a scientific fact, and you can find references stating so in every nutritional biochemistry and exercise science textbook ever published, as well as thousands of exercise science, nutrition, and obesity journal papers, which have all been through scrupulous peer review.

Anyone who claims, "You can eat as much as you want and still lose weight" is lying, perpetuating a myth, and, if stated in advertisements, breaking the law, according to the FTC. "Calories don't count" is the biggest and most harmful myth in the weight-loss industry.

Granted, strict calorie counting has limitations. Inaccurate nutrition labeling, imprecise weighing and measuring, underestimating serving sizes, and forgetting to report everything you eat all make it far from a perfect science. And that's just on the food intake side. On the expenditure side, the best you can get is a close estimate of how many calories you're actually burning.

Some people count portions instead of calories and then simply adjust portion size according to their results. This can be an effective approach, although a downside is that you're guessing at your caloric intake. If you guess right, you lose weight. If you guess wrong, you don't. Calorie counting is ideal because it increases awareness and takes out as much of the nutrition guesswork as possible.

However, it's not mandatory to know exactly how many calories you're eating as long as you understand the energy balance equation on an intellectual level and you know how to apply it practically in your daily life. Once you've established a baseline, if you want to speed up your fat loss, you simply increase your energy expenditure by getting more exercise and activity, decrease your energy intake by eating smaller portions, or both.

Many people still deny the law of calorie balance in the face of scientific evidence. Some proponents of low-carbohydrate diets are especially notorious for this. They believe that as long as you cut enough carbs, you can eat as much as you want. I assure you, if you have a maintenance level of 2,000 calories a day and you eat 4,000 calories a day of protein and fat (no carbs), you will gain fat. A lot. Fast. Like the law of gravity, the law of energy balance keeps on working whether you believe in it or not.

MYTH #2: Overweight people have a slower metabolism than thin people

Overweight people often claim that a slow metabolism is the reason they can't lose weight. This has been disproven time after time in a variety of tightly controlled experimental research trials. Believe it or not, the reverse is true.

Men and women with a large body mass actually burn more calories because their resting metabolic rate is directly linked to their total body mass and their lean body mass. Simply stated, large people burn more calories than small people. Furthermore, the energy cost of moving around a very large body is greater than the energy cost of moving a light body. Any person who doubts this should strap on a sixty-pound weighted vest or backpack, go for an uphill hike, and then judge for himself.

As you lose weight, your calorie requirements go down in proportion to your total body mass. If you keep eating the same for your smaller body as you did for your larger body, your calorie deficit shrinks as you lose weight. This not only explains in part the "slow metabolism" myth, but it also helps explain weight-loss plateaus and weight regain.

MYTH #3: Some people are diet-resistant and can't lose weight

Many people truly believe that nothing ever works for them and they're physically incapable of getting leaner. More people than I can count have told me I was their "last resort," as if they were poised to give up forever after one last try. The reasons they gave were endless: slow metabolism, bad genetics, too old, medical problems, menopause, glandular problems, or "it's just not in the cards for me."

I often joke around and say, "You have a glandular problem all right, your mouth gland is malfunctioning several times a day and you're eating too much." For some reason, not everyone finds that amusing. All kidding aside, thyroid disorders are one example of a legitimate problem that can affect metabolism and should be diagnosed and treated by a medical professional. Prader-Willi syndrome is an example of a rare chromosome defect that causes insatiable appetite and life-threatening obesity. A very rare mutation in the leptin gene could also cause severe obesity.

After rare genetic anomalies are ruled out and thyroid disorders are diagnosed and treated, could genetics, metabolism, age, hormones, or anything else really be enough to make you resistant to a low-calorie diet? In 1992 a team of researchers led by Steven Lichtman at St. Luke's–Roosevelt Hospital in New York City decided to put this common question to the test of scientific scrutiny. They set up a well-controlled clinical trial and recruited a group of subjects with a history of self-professed "diet resistance." Many of the subjects claimed they were eating only 1,200 calories a day but couldn't lose weight. Then they set up a well-controlled clinical trial to compare the "diet-resistant" group to a control group. The results were published in the prestigious *New England Journal of Medicine*.

The metabolic response and number of calories burned during exercise did not differ significantly between groups, and no subject in the "diet resistant" group had a substantially reduced resting metabolic rate. That was another nail in the coffin of the slow-metabolism myth, but the biggest surprise was how much food intake was underreported. It was shocking. The "diet-resistant" group ate 1,053 calories per day more than they reported—an underestimation of 47 percent. They also overestimated how many calories they burned by 51 percent.

The researchers concluded, "Failure to lose weight despite a self-reported low caloric intake can be explained by substantial misreporting of food intake and low physical activity." This was not an isolated finding. Underestimating food intake is not only well documented, it's actually so pervasive it creates a major challenge in dietetics and weight-loss research.

Other studies have revealed that obese people underreport more than nonobese people and women underreport more than men. "Selective underreporting" was also identified, where subjects seem to get "amnesia" about eating specific foods such as fats or sweets. Even health professionals are not immune. In a 1999 study by the *Journal of Nutrition*, "Underreporting of Habitual Food Intake in Highly Motivated Lean Women," a group of dietitians underestimated their food intake by an average of 16 percent.

The bottom line: almost all of us are terrible at guessing our caloric intake.

MYTH #4: Your genetics are why you are overweight

According to the latest research from the Human Genome Project, there's a significant genetic component to obesity. However, scientists say that severe mutations in the obesity gene are rare in humans and have raised doubts that genetics could be a direct cause of the current obesity epidemic.

Dr. Claude Bouchard of the Human Genomics Laboratory in Baton Rouge, Louisiana, suggests the following contributing factors as causes of obesity:

- physical environment;
- social environment;

- behavior;
- biology (genetics).

Dr. Bouchard says, "The obesity epidemic that we are facing today has developed only over the past fifty years and can't be explained by changes in our genome."

It's only when a genetic predisposition meets an "obesogenic environment"—where calorie-dense processed foods are readily available, activity is reduced by labor-saving devices, and a sedentary lifestyle is encouraged—that the genes express themselves. Therefore, claiming that genetics are more influential than behavior and lifestyle is completely false.

Body fat is a complex problem with numerous causes and genetics are only one part. Although many people prefer to pin all the blame on something outside their control, current evidence says that the condition your body is in today is primarily a product of your own lifestyle, social influences, behavior, and mind-set and not just genetics.

MYTH #5: Dietary fat makes you gain body fat

"The fat you eat is the fat you wear." I will never forget those words, which were written by a medical doctor in a best-selling diet book back in the 1980s. The problem was, the doctor was wrong. Dogma such as this was responsible for millions of people becoming "fat phobics."

At the peak of the low-fat diet movement, it seemed like almost every food package had the words "no fat" or "low fat" emblazoned in bold print. Even hard candies had "0% fat" printed on the packages. Well, no kidding, hard candy is 100 percent sugar. The only thing more insulting to our intelligence is when egg cartons say "low in carbs."

Why are most people so afraid of dietary fat? One simple answer is plausibility. It seems completely reasonable to assume that fat in your food will get stored as fat on your body. After all, it's the same stuff, right? It sounds believable, but it's a fallacy.

Another reason the "fat makes you fat" myth survives today is because there's research that says it does. Anyone who wants to make a case against dietary fat can pull out a whole stack of studies that show eating more fat is associated with weight gain. This is another classic case of confusing correlation with causation. The truth is, the subjects simply ate more calories, and dietary fat was the high-payload vehicle.

Dietary fat is the most calorie-dense macronutrient, with nine calories per gram, as compared to four calories per gram in carbohydrate or protein. This can be a problem if you're not careful. Since high-fat foods are high-calorie foods, people who eat more fat but don't pay attention to portion sizes tend to eat more total calories, especially in a mixed diet that contains a lot of concentrated carbohydrates, as well.

However, this still doesn't mean that eating fat causes you to gain fat. You can eat a large percentage of your calories from dietary fat, but if you're in a caloric deficit you will still lose weight. Notice how this brings us back to the calories-in versus calories-out principle. We'll keep coming back to this point. Everything comes full circle to calories.

MYTH #6: Carbohydrates make you fat

Much of what I said about dietary fat applies to carbs as well. If you choose, you can eat a fairly generous proportion of your calories from carbs and lose weight, as long as you stay in a calorie deficit.

If this is true, then why are low-carbohydrate diets so popular? It's probably because they work quite well for many people. Low-carb diets may have an advantage for weight loss, although it may not be what you've been led to believe. Low-carb diets help to control calories automatically and they may be better at controlling appetite. If the low-carb diet is also high in protein, this may be a further advantage because you expend more calories digesting protein.

It's easy to overeat sugars, starchy carbs, and grains, but it's difficult to overeat when you restrict an entire group of calorie-dense foods. If I told you the only thing you could eat was lean proteins like chicken breast, fish, egg whites, some healthy fats, green vegetables, and salad vegetables, it would be nearly impossible to overeat. In dietetics this is often referred to as "stimulus narrowing," where limiting the food choices increases compliance to a caloric deficit.

Low-carb diet books often claim, "Eat all you want and lose weight," but by giving you some strict rules about which foods you can and cannot eat, they have tricked you into eating less. Some dietitians like to say low-carb diets are low-calorie diets in disguise. I'm not saying that's a bad thing. If the foods you choose make you feel fuller on fewer calories so you eat less overall, I'd call that a virtue. It only becomes a negative if you begin to believe that "calories don't count" or "carbs are evil," and especially if you fail to distinguish between nutrient-dense natural carbs and nutrient-sparse processed carbs.

MYTH #7: Dietary changes for health and weight loss are one and the same

There's a big difference between nutrient density and calorie density of various foods. There's also a big difference between the health benefits and body composition benefits you get from eating certain foods. I call this the health–body fat paradox.

High body fat usually comes with a cluster of other health problems, including hypertension, type 2 diabetes, high cholesterol, high blood sugar, and high triglycerides. However, the first part of the health–body fat paradox is that you can be healthy while having unwanted excess body fat, and you can be lean while having health problems. The ideal is lean and healthy, not one or the other.

The second part of the paradox is that you could eat white sugar, white flour, or virtually any other junk food you can think of, and if you consume only small amounts so you stay in a caloric deficit, you'll still lose body fat. Conversely, you can be a clean-eating fanatic and cut 100 percent of the refined foods out of your diet, and while you'll get health benefits from that, if you're in a calorie surplus, you'll still gain body fat.

Weight gain or loss is dictated primarily by calorie quantity. Health is dictated primarily by calorie quality. The ideal is the right combination of calorie quantity and calorie quality, not one or the other. When you understand the health—body fat paradox, you'll be able to strike the right balance between calorie quality and calorie quantity. You'll also understand when a recommendation is made for health purposes as compared to weight-loss purposes. They usually overlap, but they're not always the same.

MYTH #8: Insulin or insulin resistance causes obesity

Insulin is a hormone your pancreas releases that's best known for regulating blood sugar and transporting glucose into your cells. Insulin also plays a role in the body fat picture because high insulin levels prevent your body from releasing fat. Insulin is also a storage hormone that carries glucose into your fat cells.

This might sound like insulin is bad news. In the low-carb world, it has become somewhat of a rallying cry that, since eating carbs causes a large release of insulin, this means "insulin makes you fat." Some authors of low-carb books have gone as far as calling insulin a "monster hormone." As with many areas of human physiology and nutrition, it's not quite that simple.

Insulin does not necessarily cause obesity, although controlling insulin should be a goal of any healthy body-fat-reducing nutrition program. Insulin is a double-edged sword you must manage carefully, but it's not some "evil fat-storing monster." Insulin is actually a very important anabolic hormone that is also responsible for transporting amino acids and glucose into muscle tissue.

For certain genetically predisposed individuals, a high-carb diet might not be the healthiest choice because it may elevate insulin levels and aggravate metabolic syndrome. Metabolic syndrome is a cluster of symptoms including high blood pressure, high triglycerides, low HDL cholesterol, high fasting blood sugar, and abdominal body fat. Metabolic syndrome is considered a prediabetic state and it can be the beginning of more serious health problems. Some experts recommend a lower-carb, higher-fat diet to help mitigate the symptoms of metabolic syndrome. It's important to remember, however, that a reduced-carb diet is often a health recommendation for managing insulin, blood sugar, and metabolic syndrome and not for weight loss per se.

Failing to make this distinction has led to many myths about the role of in-

sulin in weight loss. Gerald Reaven, the Stanford diabetes researcher who literally wrote the book on metabolic syndrome (*Syndrome* X), said that insulin does
not make you gain weight and neither does insulin resistance. In fact, he said,
"the notion is almost ludicrous." As he explained:

> YEARS AGO, WE PUT PEOPLE with different degrees of the insulin resistance on
> dramatically different diets. In one study, carbohydrates were either 85 or 17 percent
> of calories. The only thing that affected their weight was how many calories they ate.
> There's not one shred of evidence that insulin resistance causes obesity. Insulin re-
> sistance means that insulin isn't acting correctly. So if you don't have enough insulin
> or if your cells aren't responding to insulin, you can't deposit glucose into cells. If
> anything, you would lose weight.

There's a close relationship between excess body fat, insulin, and metabolic
syndrome, and losing weight will improve your health. It's the surplus of calories, however, that actually causes the fat gain, and it always takes a calorie
deficit to lose it.

Be Careful: Cause and Effect Can Be Tricky

You may have had some success in losing weight in the past, but do you understand why? These myths and the reasons we believe them tell us one thing: we
must be careful in interpreting how our results were achieved. Misunderstanding cause and effect can lead you to believe in myths and even downright
weird stuff.

It's easy to attribute weight loss or lack of weight loss to one thing when it
was really caused by something different altogether. On the surface it seems to
make total sense that A occurred, then B occurred, therefore A caused B. For
example, we take a fat-burning pill and suddenly begin losing weight, therefore
we believe the cause of our weight loss was the fat-burning pill.

This fails to account for the fact that we tend to make health changes in clus-
ters and other things may have caused or contributed to the weight loss. If we

take fat-burning pills when starting a diet and exercise program, we tend to credit the pill with the results rather than the increased activity or improved eating habits.

In this chapter, you've begun practicing important new habits of critical thinking and you've started clearing your mind of the fallacies and myths that may have held you back in the past. The next step in setting the stage is to learn what new beliefs and attitudes to put in the mental space you just created now that you've tossed the old myths and limiting beliefs in the trash.

Attitudes and Beliefs That Set the Stage for Success

CHAPTER THREE

> WHEN you change the way you look at things, the things you look at change.
>
> —DR. WAYNE DYER

Just tell me what to *do*!" It's the plea I've heard from virtually every person I've met in a consultation. "What foods should I eat?" and "What workout should I do?" are the most common first questions. I don't think any new client has ever walked into my office and said, "Tell me what to think," or "Tell me what to believe." Those would be odd questions to ask a fitness coach, I suppose, but that's actually a shame because it's not your nutrition or workout that makes or breaks you.

43

There are hundreds of different exercise programs to choose from and any one of them can work if they're grounded in a few basic principles of exercise science. There are dozens of valid approaches to nutrition as well. As long as there's a calorie deficit, any diet can cause weight loss.

I'm not suggesting that nutrition and training strategies aren't important. If you don't work smart, you can work harder than anyone and still get no results. On the other hand, two people could use the same effective strategy and one will succeed while the other will fail. If you want to know the difference between the two of them, then don't stop at asking what diet or workout program to follow. The most important question is *what makes you follow your program?*

What makes you take action? Where does motivation come from? Why do some people persist and others quit? What triggers impulsive behaviors? What causes someone to sabotage a perfectly good plan? All the answers are in the mind. You never take an action without first thinking a thought. If it's not a conscious thought, then it's an unconscious one, but a neural impulse always comes first.

I've spent more than twenty years picking the brains of lean people. Naturally, I'm interested in what they eat and how they train, but as a student of psychology as well as physiology, I'm equally interested in how they think. Sometimes you can pick up what's going on inside someone's head by listening to what they say. But it's not always that easy because most mental processes take place on the unconscious level. Usually it takes some digging to bring a person's mental strategies to the surface.

One of my greatest discoveries is that successful people share similar attitudes and beliefs, and that these thought patterns can be learned and duplicated. That's an exciting prospect. It means that if you learn to think like a lean person, you'll increase your chances of becoming one.

Attitude: Perception Is Reality

An attitude is your perspective or unique way of looking at things. The world out there is the same, but every person experiences it differently through his own filters of perception. Your attitude is like a lens that determines how you see events, circumstances, yourself, and other people. Some people see things through rose-colored "optimism glasses," while others see things through dark and gloomy "pessimism glasses."

Most people allow their present results and circumstances to control their attitude. They look at the scale, and their attitude reflects what the scale says. If their weight is down, their attitude is positive. If their weight is up, their attitude is negative. They look in the mirror and if they like what they see, they're happy. If they don't, they're not. It never occurs to them that attitude is an inside job. Attitude is a choice.

Anybody can be positive when the results are good, but successful people choose a positive attitude when it counts the most—in the face of difficulty. No matter what the scale says, it doesn't bother them because they know it's only feedback. When they look in the mirror, instead of seeing what's reflected, they visualize their bodies the way they want them to look. This is a simple shift in thinking, but it's not easy to do. If you can master it, the future is yours to create.

Changing your attitude is a simple matter of changing the way you look at things. Zooming in on the details, getting the big, panoramic picture, or seeing things from the other side can sometimes change everything. The name for this is reframing, a technique that comes from the field of Neuro-Linguistic Programming (NLP). Reframing also includes when you attach a new meaning to life's events. Sometimes it's as simple as changing a single word.

Reframing with Words

Changing the words you use can change the way you think, feel, and act. Words can help or hurt, motivate or discourage, build or destroy. In fact, words can physically affect your body as well as your mind. Howard Fields, M.D., a neurobiologist and professor at the University of California, San Francisco, explains that the words of a doctor can affect a patient's health.

IT'S VERY IMPORTANT for people to know that words can powerfully affect their brains in ways that are beneficial or harmful. If you tell people things that are negative about a medication, or if you communicate by body language or tone of voice that you really don't think something is going to work, but, "Oh well, let's try it," then that can actually reduce the effectiveness of a powerful analgesic.

Healthy and successful people have their own vocabulary. They see problems as challenges. They view failure as feedback. Frustration is fascination. Confused means curious. Shoulds become musts. Older means wiser. An injury is an inconvenience. These are all powerful one-word reframes.

The fittest people I know see "plateaus" as a signal to change their workouts. The unfit see plateaus as a signal to quit. Unfit people say they have to work out. Fit people say they get to work out. To the former, exercise is chore. To the latter, exercise is an opportunity to improve and they feel grateful for it, because they know other people are not as physically blessed as they are.

"Diet" is a word worth reframing because it's semantically loaded yet ambiguous. To most people it has negative connotations, including deprivation, hunger, and bland foods. A diet is seen as a restrictive eating program that you go on, suffer through, and then go off. I prefer "nutrition program" instead of "diet." This removes emotional baggage, implies structure, and presumes you'll be eating nutrient-dense food.

"Loser" is another word that must go. No one likes to experience a sense of loss and people who are success-oriented won't let themselves become labeled as losers. If you're a winner and you tell yourself you're going to lose some weight, your brain says, "You don't want to lose anything," so you unconsciously eat more or skip your workouts to make sure you don't lose. Instead of losing fat, try burning, incinerating, releasing, shedding, or discarding fat. While you're at it, don't quit anything. Just stop. No one likes a quitter.

The word "can't" does not mean something is impossible. It means you can choose not to do it. "Can't" really means that you won't or you haven't yet. When you use the word "can't," it completely stops your brain from working on solutions. To move your brain into a possibilities frame, change "I can't" into "How can I?" It's not that you can't, you merely haven't figured out how yet.

Reframing Meanings

The American inventor Thomas Edison labored for years to find a filament that would burn in the incandescent lightbulb. On October 22, 1879, after thousands of unsuccessful experiments, Edison finally discovered the right carbon filament and created the world's first practical electric lightbulb. When reporters asked what it felt like to fail so many times, Edison said, "I didn't fail, I found more than ten thousand ways that won't work. Every wrong attempt discarded was another step forward."

This is one of the most brilliant and famous reframes in history. Had Edison not chosen to view each failed experiment as a learning experience that brought him one step closer to success, he never would have persisted and who knows how much longer we would have been lighting candles. A simple reframe in meaning or perspective can keep you forging ahead through adversity where others would quit.

Failure is not a person, it's an event. Before he succeeded, Edison never thought of himself as a failure. It was the experiments that failed. Failure can be a learning experience and a source of valuable feedback. It can even be a blessing in disguise. The failure to achieve a desired result has nothing to do with you as a person. It means that the strategy you used was a poor one or it was an effective strategy that you didn't apply consistently.

How do you perceive failures, problems, or obstacles? Think about it, then ask questions such as these:

- How could I look at this from a different perspective?
- What different meaning could I give to this?
- What's the hidden benefit in this?
- What can I learn from this?

Reframing to Eliminate Excuses and Resolve Inner Conflicts

Have you ever felt like your attempts at getting leaner were like having one foot on the brake and one foot on the gas? If so, then opposing desires inside your mind may have created an internal conflict. You may want nothing more than a lean, healthy body, but dieting means deprivation to you. You also want to be fit, strong, and muscular, but exercise means pain to you. Part of you wants the pleasure of a better body, but another part wants to avoid the discomfort of getting there.

Inner conflicts often show up in the form of procrastination or self-sabotage, which are then rationalized away with excuses. In reality, excuses are simply habitual ways of thinking that you've never challenged. If people were as creative in coming up with solutions as they were in coming up with excuses, there would be a lot fewer problems in the world.

Reframing can help you eliminate excuses by shifting your thoughts toward personal responsibility, possibility, choice, and win-win scenarios. If you get creative with reframing, you may find yourself laughing, because old excuses start to look ridiculous. Here are some great examples.

Conflict: I have no time.
Solution: You have all the time there is—twenty-four hours a day—the same amount as Bill Gates, Richard Branson, and Warren Buffett. It's not that you don't have enough time, you simply haven't chosen your priorities or put them in the proper order yet.

Conflict: I have to give up all the foods I love.
Solution: Where did you get that idea? You can eat chocolate, ice cream, pizza, or whatever else you want as long as you eat those foods infrequently and in small amounts. The only thing you have to give up is eating more calories than you need.

Conflict: I'll never lose weight because of my genetics.
Solution: Genetics do not stop you from losing weight unless a genetic predis-

position meets a sedentary lifestyle and unsupportive environment. You simply haven't made all the necessary improvements to your environment and lifestyle yet.

Conflict: Life is too short to be in the gym all the time.
Solution: Your life will be really short if you don't take care of your health. Who said you had to be in the gym all the time? Maybe you just haven't learned how to train in a time-efficient manner yet. You can save time by training at home.

Conflict: I have to take care of others first.
Solution: You can take care of yourself *and* others: it's not an either/or situation. And if you don't take care of yourself first, you can't take care of others.

Conflict: If I go on a diet I'll never be able to eat at restaurants.
Solution: Never? That's ridiculous. If you choose, you can eat healthy in almost any restaurant. You simply need to make good choices and keep the portions small.

Conflict: If I work out every day then I won't have any social life.
Solution: What a silly idea. Exercise can be one of the biggest parts of your social life. You can recruit a friend to work out with you and support each other. If you go to a gym, that's a great place to meet people.

Conflict: It's impossible for me to start a workout program now because I have a bad (insert your excuse: knee, shoulder, back, etc.).
Solution: Impossible or just a bit more challenging? Having an injury doesn't mean you can't do anything, it means that you'll need to work around it and focus on what you *can* do. Besides, even if you were laid up in bed, you can still get leaner and healthier by improving your nutrition.

Now you have some new perspectives to experiment with. The next time you catch a spell of excusitis or full-blown it's-not-my-fault disease, or whenever that negative internal voice spouts off inside your head, you can interrupt that inner critic and challenge those old ways of thinking. Be like Edison and remind yourself that most events are not inherently good or bad, it all depends on how you look at them.

The Miraculous Power of Belief

At the Baylor College of Medicine in Houston, Dr. Bruce Mosley had been successfully performing arthroscopic knee surgeries for years using two different procedures. The problem was, he didn't know which one was more effective, so he petitioned a colleague, Dr. Nelda Wray, for advice on how to conduct a study that would single out the better technique. To his surprise, she advised him that comparing the two surgeries wouldn't work. What he needed was a placebo study. Dr. Mosley almost burst out laughing at the idea of doing sham surgery, but later decided to proceed. What happened made medical history.

The patients were divided into three groups. In group one, the subjects received the first procedure, which consisted of washing out the inside of the knee joint. In group two, the procedure also smoothed out the rough cartilage surfaces. Group three included two war veterans, Tim Perez and Sylvester Colligan, who both suffered from crippling knee pain. Dr. Mosley administered anesthesia and made three incisions as he did with the other procedures. Then he literally faked the rest of the surgery. After forty minutes, he sewed up the cuts, having done absolutely nothing to his patient's knees.

The astonishing results were published in the *New England Journal of Medicine* in July 2002. All three groups experienced the same outcome: they improved and recovered. Dr. Mosley concluded that the results of *all three* surgeries may have been due to the placebo effect, a phenomenon usually triggered when test subjects get well after taking a pill that contains no actual medication. Sylvester Colligan can now walk. Tim Perez plays basketball with his grandchildren. "In this world, anything is possible when you put your mind to it," said Perez. "Your mind can work miracles."

What Are Beliefs?

Belief is the power behind the placebo effect. But this mental power is not seen only in dramatic placebo studies and rare cases of spontaneous healing. Your beliefs work for or against you daily in every area of your life. Beliefs are not only involved directly in the mind-body connection, they're also unconscious programs that control your behavior. Empowering beliefs can be a force that drives you to success beyond your wildest dreams. Limiting beliefs, however, can put a cap on your level of achievement, stop you from taking action, or sabotage the best plans.

Beliefs are not facts. They're only interpretations or value judgments you make about yourself, your experiences, and the world around you. Think of beliefs as mental software installed in your brain that takes in raw data through your senses and then applies meaning to it.

If you weighed yourself and said, "My weight hasn't changed this week," it would be a verifiable fact. But if you continued, "That means this diet doesn't work and I'll never lose weight," those would not be facts. You created beliefs about what you thought your results meant, but your interpretations may have been incorrect. Your nutrition plan could be very effective, but you might have underestimated how much you were eating. You might have gained water weight or grown new muscle tissue, masking weight loss.

You learned in the last chapter how easy it can be to believe myths about weight loss and body fat. You formed these beliefs through erroneous thinking or accepted them from authorities, the media, your parents, and your peers. In the same way, you may have formed many other beliefs that might not be true. You have beliefs about your environment, your behaviors, your capabilities, and even your identity. Once you form a belief, you'll act as though it's true and you'll tend to resist or filter out anything that disagrees with it. When it comes to diet and nutrition, many people believe in things with an almost religious conviction.

Low-carb diets, for example, have legitimate fat-loss benefits such as decreasing appetite and controlling insulin. Unfortunately, when someone is successful with a low-carb diet, they often take on dogmatic and inaccurate beliefs. For the rest of their lives, they might look at almost all carbohydrates as fattening, and since they counted carbs, not calories, they often think that calories don't count, a dangerous and false belief. But try convincing a formerly obese low-carb dieter of that (it's about as easy as getting them to change their religion). By the way, if you're a successful high-carb/low-fat dieter, don't gloat too much, because mistaken beliefs about high-carb/low-fat diets are just as common.

Some beliefs are much stronger than others. With the possible exception of spiritual beliefs, identity beliefs are the strongest of all. You can spot a belief about your identity by what you say after "I am." "I am an overeater" is an identity belief. If you said, "I overeat occasionally," that's not as strong because you'd be talking about a behavior, not a person, and a behavior is easier to change than a person.

Beliefs about your values are also high on the hierarchy and can be extremely influential because your values represent what's most important to you. If you believe that health is your greatest form of wealth and it's the most important priority in your life, it will have a massive impact on how you act.

Beliefs should be honored and respected, but they should also be scrutinized carefully. A belief is only a generalization or evaluation in your mind. If you accept the possibility that you might believe things that are actually holding you back, then you've taken the first step toward transforming your behavior, your body, and your life.

How Beliefs Affect Your Behavior and Play Out in Your Life

If you don't believe something is possible, you usually won't attempt it. If you try while your mind is preoccupied with doubts, you won't perform well and you're likely to quit at the first obstacle.

I've seen this happen numerous times during body transformation competitions. With exotic vacations or thousands of dollars in prize money dangled as incentives, these contests have become immensely popular and you'd think they would provide all the motivation you'd need to achieve the best shape of your life. The attrition statistics tell a different story. Most people who enter these contests never finish.

After working with many of the dropouts, I discovered that while they started with good intentions and good nutrition and training strategies, unconsciously, they didn't believe they could achieve a ripped body worthy of an "after" photograph. Because their new goal was inconsistent with their old mental programming, they sabotaged their diet or gave up at the first rough patch.

My solution was to show them examples of other people just like them, or worse off than them, who successfully completed the challenge. Then I helped them reprogram their self-image. In some cases, I didn't change a thing in their nutrition and training. Simply working on their mental strategies removed the unconscious blocks to executing their behavioral strategies.

People may say they believe in something, but that's their conscious mind speaking. Behavior is the true expression of what people believe on the unconscious level. People don't always do what they say, but they always do what they believe.

What you believe is possible and what you believe you're capable of will affect what endeavors you attempt and whether you persist through adversity or give up. What you believe will affect every behavior and decision you make each day. Some people won't eat certain foods because of their religious beliefs. Some people don't eat meat because they believe it's unethical to kill animals. I know folks who believe that artificial sweeteners are poison, so they won't touch them.

If you can fit a certain behavior into your belief system, it will be easy to do. If you strongly value your health, and if you believe that eating fruits and vegetables will give you unbounded energy and vitality, then you won't have to force yourself to eat them—you'll crave them.

If doing something violates your values and beliefs, it will be out of the question. Your nervous system will literally short-circuit your behavior before you can do it. If you believe that white flour and white sugar are toxic substances that will slowly poison you, then you won't have to use willpower to stay away from them—you'll be repulsed by them.

How to Identify Limiting Beliefs

Some beliefs are part of your conscious awareness, but the beliefs that limit you most are usually ones you don't know you have. Even if you follow an effective training and nutrition strategy, limiting beliefs operating below the surface will lead to self-sabotage. Limiting beliefs must be dug up, ripped out, and replaced, because only then have you dealt with the true cause of many body fat problems at the source.

Flushing out limiting beliefs takes honest self-analysis. Start by asking yourself these questions:

- What causes me to be overweight?
- What's preventing me from getting leaner?

If you listen carefully to your answers, you may hear limiting beliefs stated as cause-and-effect or if-then relationships. For example:

"I'm overweight and can't get leaner because . . ."

- I have no motivation.
- I have no willpower.
- I have a slow metabolism.
- I hate exercise.
- I love food.
- I'm injured.
- I overeat when I'm stressed.
- I don't know what to eat or how to cook.
- If you're over fifty, then it's too late.
- If I have one bite, then I can't stop.

- If you have kids and a job, then there's no time to work out.
- If I try and fail, then I'll hate myself.

One dead giveaway of limiting beliefs is use of all-or-none words such as "always" or "never." Limiting beliefs also show up with the words "can't" or "impossible":

- I'll never see my abs.
- I always gain back the weight.
- You can't lose weight if you have a thyroid problem.
- It's impossible to wear the jeans size I wore when I was twenty-one.

Challenging and Weakening the Old Limiting Beliefs

Limiting beliefs include any excuse that's holding you back or any thought preventing you from taking action. Once you've identified a limiting belief, the next step is to challenge it. Strong beliefs are not always easy to get rid of. However, even with deeply held beliefs, the challenge process can weaken them. By questioning your old beliefs, you create a doubt, and that's all the opening you need to slip an empowering new belief in its place.

Challenge the Belief Directly

The first way to break down a limiting belief is to question its validity. Put that belief on the witness stand and "cross-examine" it as if you were a prosecuting attorney in a courtroom. Find evidence against it, build your case, and prove that it's not true.

"I'm too old" is an excuse I have to put on trial often now that the baby boomer generation makes up the largest part of the population. In my first consultation with Bill, a fifty-year-old coaching client, it took less than five minutes to get him to deliver a "not true" verdict on his own self-limiting belief. Bill arrived in my office expecting it to be "impossible" to be in the shape he was in at age twenty. That's when I started my questioning: How do you know that? Is it impossible or just a little harder? How do you explain that thousands of fifty-plus-year-olds have gotten so fit and lean? If other fifty-year-olds like you have done it, then what's stopping you?

Then I flipped through a three-ring binder of testimonials and case studies. Right before his eyes were pages of photographs of fifty- and even sixty-year-olds with no abs in sight before and six-pack abs after. Bill left our meeting that day no longer believing that it was impossible.

Challenge the Belief by Questioning the Source

In the previous chapter, you learned that to avoid becoming a victim of fitness myths and fat-burning fraud, you must question everything, including where you got your information. To avoid becoming a victim of your own limiting beliefs, you must do the same thing and challenge them by questioning the source. Did you choose them or were they handed down from authorities, parents, or friends? Have you been living your entire life based on someone else's belief system? Sometimes the mere realization that a belief is not yours is enough to destroy it.

Challenge the Usefulness of the Belief

Throughout your life, you picked up beliefs that never served you, but you've held on to them ever since. You also adopted beliefs that served you at one time, such as during childhood, but they lost their usefulness long ago. If you don't believe in Santa Claus or the tooth fairy anymore, then why hold on to other beliefs you've outgrown? You must constantly analyze your beliefs to see if they still have or ever had any utility. Ask yourself: Does this belief serve any useful purpose? Has this belief ever kept me from getting something I wanted? Does this belief help me or hurt me? If this belief hurts me, limits me, serves no useful purpose, or keeps me from getting what I want, then how quickly can I get rid of it?

Motivation doesn't come only from rewards and benefits (the carrot). For many people, pain or consequence (the stick) is an even greater motivator. Understanding consequences can be the final nail in the coffin of old limiting beliefs. When you think of a belief that's limiting you, ask yourself: What are the consequences of keeping it? What has this cost me in the past? What is it costing me today? What will be the future consequences if I don't change this now?

Installing New Success Beliefs

You weren't born with any beliefs; you acquired and developed all of them over time. This means you can change an old belief or acquire a new one anytime you choose. This does not imply that you can simply challenge the belief and you'll be home free. The famous aphorism "Nature abhors a vacuum" is remarkably true of the human mind. When you remove an old belief, it creates a void that begs to be filled. That's why you must choose and install a new belief to take the place of the old one.

Imagine that you could go to the store and buy any belief you wanted, as if it were a piece of software, which you could take home and download onto your computer. Well, you can, metaphorically speaking. That computer is your brain and it's ready and waiting to accept any new programs you choose. So ask yourself what beliefs would be most useful for you to install in your mental computer.

Seven Essential Success Attitudes and Beliefs That Make Change Possible

I could go on for pages listing the success beliefs of lean people that would be useful for you to emulate. There's a bigger picture, however, that's a much higher priority for you at this point. What would happen if you believed that nothing ever worked for you or you simply weren't able to lose weight? What if you thought it would be nice to slim down, but it wasn't that important to you at the moment? What if you were indifferent? These types of negative attitudes and beliefs would override and sabotage all the others beneath them. That's why the best way to start reprogramming your mind is to focus on the higher-level beliefs and consider them the essentials or prerequisites for your success. These are the beliefs that make change possible.

#1: POSSIBILITY: It's Achievable

Just as you must open yourself to doubt your old limiting beliefs, you must open yourself to believe your new goals are possible. I recently read a story about an entrepreneur who built his small business into a $500 million corporation from scratch in just thirty-six months. In an interview, the thirty-seven-year-old businessman said, "Making a million dollars was the easiest thing I ever did. Believing it could happen to me was the hard part. That took thirty-seven years."

Achieving huge goals in the physical sense always requires work, but it sometimes isn't as difficult as you think. Achieving it first in the mind is the hard part. The question is, do you believe you can do it? When you believe something is possible, you act as if it's possible. When you don't believe it's possible, you act as if it's impossible. If you're going to act as if something is impossible, then act as though it's impossible to fail.

When I was a teenager just starting to lift weights, they told me it was impossible to be a top bodybuilder without taking steroids. I chose to believe differently. What made it possible is that I looked for role models. I found people I knew were natural who had amazing bodies. The nonbelievers said, "No way. They're lying. They're cheating. They're on 'roids!" They set limitations on themselves by choosing that belief. I looked for champion drug-free athletes and said, "They did, so I can do it too." With that belief, I went on to do "the impossible" by winning numerous bodybuilding championships, and today I have more than two dozen trophies to show for it.

Experts said it was impossible to run a mile in under four minutes until Roger Bannister did it in 1954. It's now the standard for all professional middle-distance runners. What made this possible? The human body didn't change. The laws of physics didn't change. It was beliefs that changed. The barrier Bannister broke was mental and once it was broken, others quickly followed.

Finding role models in your area of endeavor is a great way to learn from the experience of others. It's also a powerful approach to belief-building. If other people like you have done it, and you've seen proof with your own eyes, then this means you know it's possible. I also suggest you look for role models who are record-breakers—explorers, visionaries, and inventors. Their examples remind you that just because something has never been done before doesn't mean it can't be done.

#2: CAPABILITY: I Am Able

Possibility is when you believe something can be done. Capability is when you believe something can be done *by you*. Finding role models is a powerful tool for changing beliefs, but in some cases, it's not enough. Some people can see a thousand examples of others who achieved a goal, but say, "Well, they can do it, but I can't."

Doubts occur if you have no references or proof to support what you want to believe. Beliefs are strengthened when you put legs of proof underneath them, like legs of a table. The more evidence you have holding up your belief, the stronger it will be.

To help boost belief in yourself, first search your past experience. Think of a time when you had a goal you didn't believe was possible, but you achieved it anyway. It might be an academic or intellectual achievement. It might be in sports. It might be a creative endeavor. It might be a successful relationship. Even if it was far removed from health or fitness goals, it's proof that you have the ability to achieve things you once thought you weren't capable of achieving.

Second, begin to gather new evidence by taking action on your fitness plan and starting to accumulate small victories. Keep your big goals in mind, but set a lot of short-term goals as well. Choose simple things you're confident you can easily achieve. For example, set a goal to go to the gym today and do a certain number of exercises, sets, and repetitions. After you've done it, write it down in a victory journal, then repeat the process and raise the bar a little higher each time.

With a small list of achieved goals and personal bests, your level of belief in yourself will increase. As you become more confident, set larger goals that you're not quite sure you can achieve yet, but they're challenges you're willing to tackle. When you start to hit those goals, your belief in yourself will skyrocket.

#3: NECESSITY: I Must Achieve It

Possibility means you believe it can be done. Capability means you believe it can be done by you. Necessity means you must do it now or else.

People will usually stay the same until the pain of staying the same becomes greater than the pain of changing. When you're dissatisfied, eventually that feeling builds up until it reaches a threshold. That's the point where pain and consequences have piled up so high that one triggering event becomes the straw that breaks the camel's back. "I'm not going to take it anymore!" "Enough is enough!" These are the types of exclamations you hear when someone has crossed the threshold and that's when they start taking massive action.

You don't have to hit rock bottom or have a health crisis to trigger a change. All you need to do is stop saying, "I should . . ." and keep asking yourself, "Why is getting leaner and reaching my health and fitness goals an absolute must right now?" The more reasons you come up with, the more likely you'll be to trigger the change. When shoulds turn into musts, then you know you've crossed the threshold of necessity.

#4: WORTHINESS: I Deserve It

Most people are unsatisfied with their bodies. This is perfectly normal. The desire to better one's circumstances is hardwired into every human being. But never confuse the desire for improvement with the belief that you're not good enough the way you are. The problem is, disliking your body can turn into disliking yourself. Disliking yourself turns into low self-worth, which means you believe you don't deserve good things in life, including a lean and healthy body. Low self-worth easily leads to apathy, depression, or self-sabotage.

Body fat is not a person, it's a temporary condition. The way your body looks today has nothing to do with your capabilities or intrinsic worth as a person. No price tag can ever be placed on your value. The capacity of your brain to learn is virtually infinite. Your creative ability is boundless. Your body is capable of astonishing feats. You have more potential than you can dream of. Most of all, you are unique. No one else has all the qualities, talents, and abilities that you possess. Your gift to yourself, the world, and your creator is to discover them, develop them, use them, and share them.

I don't think you can feel your best if you're not engaged in the journey of self-improvement. Unfulfilled potential inside of you will always call out in the form of a longing, desire, or sense of dissatisfaction. If you're not doing anything, don't be surprised if you feel unworthy of receiving anything. It's the process of improvement and creation that makes you feel good about yourself, more than the end result.

If you get moving and take some small steps with a good action strategy, you'll immediately feel better about yourself because you'll know you're improving yourself. Even if you don't notice the small body changes that happen from one workout to the next, you'll feel better just by taking a step in the right direction. Action cures a lot of problems.

#5: DESIRE: I Want It

When you say, "I want this," it's a statement of desire. How badly you want something depends on how important it is to you. Everything on the important list in your life is called a value and values are among the most powerful beliefs. You literally organize your entire life around them. What's most and least important to you influences how you spend your time and sets the boundaries and standards for your behaviors. If you want to know your values, simply ask: What's most important to me in life? What's most important to me about being healthy? What's most important to me about having a lean body?

If you're not clear about your values and you lack strong reasons why you must get healthy, lean, and fit, this will manifest in lack of desire, low motivation, or neglect. When it's time to work out, you'll find something else you need to do, and ironically, you'll probably say you never have time to exercise.

Unfortunately, exercise and nutrition usually aren't very high on most people's values list. It often takes some kind of health crisis before they're forced to make them a priority. If health and fitness aren't high on your list yet, remind yourself that everything else you value in life, including your family, finances, and career success, depends on you being in good health.

#6: EXPECTATION: I Expect It

Physicians and psychologists say that expectancy is the power behind the placebo effect. If a suffering person is given a sugar pill and they're congruently told by a respected doctor that it's a powerful new painkiller, the patient gets immediate relief, even if the pill was an inert substance. The belief in the physician and the pill along with the expectation of a positive result activates forces in the mind that physically affect the body.

Expectation is when you believe that if you follow a strategy or plan, then as sure as the sun will rise tomorrow, you'll get the results you want. You feel expectation as a powerful sense of certainty. When you decisively choose a strategy and you're confident that your strategy will work, your level of expectancy rises. When you take action and expect success, you almost always achieve it.

#7: WILLINGNESS: I Am Willing

Ultimately, your success will be a measure of how willing you are to do what it takes. Personal development programs claiming to help you reach your goals have become a part of popular culture today, and I think that's a good thing. We can shortcut our learning curve by finding and learning from mentors. Unfortunately, the desire to get something for nothing is so pervasive, it has even infected the self-help industry. We're promised health, wealth, and happiness with positive thinking, visualization, or meditation alone. Sometimes we're told that all we have to do is pop in a CD, sit back, listen, and our brain will be programmed for success.

Positive thoughts, images, and feelings are beneficial to the degree that they help stimulate action. The mind-body connection is an exciting new frontier that we're just beginning to understand, but believing you can "think yourself thin" is wishful thinking. As motivational speaker Jim Rohn cautions, "Affirmation without action is the beginning of delusion." The mind can affect the body directly, as the placebo effect demonstrates, but we must take an active role in creating change.

There's a huge difference between wishing and willing. Almost every person on earth would like lots of money, a nice home, great relationships, perfect health, and a lean body. But not many are willing to do what it takes to get them. When you once believed you had no time to train but you now get up an hour earlier every morning without complaining because it's the only time you have to exercise given your work and family commitments, then you know you're willing. When you're willing to do whatever it takes, you're ready to receive whatever you want.

Change Can Happen in an Instant

Simply by reading this chapter, some of your attitudes and beliefs may have already begun to change. By shifting your perspective and bringing limiting beliefs out of the unconscious into the conscious level, this increase in personal awareness is often enough to initiate some amazing changes.

Although some mental changes take time—and major physical changes always take time—belief change can happen in an instant. You can stop believing in a falsehood the second a truth enters your awareness. One new experience can change your view of the world. One question can lead to a solution. One new fact or piece of evidence can change a belief.

Now that your mind is open to this possibility, you're ready for the fourth and final phase necessary to set the stage for your success: freeing yourself from emotional eating.

Freedom from Emotional Eating

I AM convinced that after diets, emotional eating is the number-one cause of obesity in the world. Many times people eat because they're bored, or lonely or miserable or tired or any one of a hundred emotional reasons, none of which has anything to do with physical hunger.

—PAUL McKENNA, HYPNOTHERAPIST

You need food for fuel, for nourishment, and as the raw material for building your muscles, tissues, and cells. However, you probably use food for many reasons outside these physical needs. No doubt, food is the centerpiece of many of your favorite social gatherings. You also might use food as a quick and easy way to feel better when you're feeling down. You may even associate food with love, warmth, caring, nurturing, and family, at least on an unconscious level.

Denying yourself completely the positive feelings and social benefits that

65

food can provide is counterproductive in the long term. My guess is that you want to be lean and happy, not lean and miserable. That's why I'm not going to ask you to completely give up any of your favorite foods or become a social outcast. In the Body Fat Solution program, we don't make all-or-none rules such as "You must follow the program 100 percent or not at all" or "You can never eat ice cream again."

It's important to allow yourself enough lenience so you don't feel deprived, but demand enough compliance so you get the results you want. Using food for nonphysical reasons only becomes a problem when you do it as a way to cope with stress or negative emotions and you do it frequently or unconsciously.

Some authorities make the subject of emotional eating sound so deep, you'd think it would take years of psychotherapy to overcome. I don't believe emotional eating is complex at all. It's a very simple problem revolving around three primary issues:

1. You eat mindlessly and impulsively, without thinking first.
2. You eat for reasons other than your physiological needs.
3. You hold beliefs about food that don't advance you toward your goals.

The heart of the matter is that you sometimes eat for the wrong reasons and you might not even realize it.

Why You Eat When You're Not Physically Hungry

Many people are under the misconception that emotional eating only happens in response to stress and to cope with negative emotions such as sadness, loneliness, disappointment, or grief. However, people eat for many other reasons that have nothing to do with physiological needs, including:

- to alleviate boredom;
- to socialize;
- to recapture a feeling or memory;

- to celebrate a special occasion;
- to fill a void or missing need;
- to feel good;
- to feel safe;
- to feel comforted;
- as a reward;
- out of habit or ritual (for example, bedtime snacking and eating in front of the TV).

Sometimes eating for nonphysical reasons is perfectly appropriate, especially for family get-togethers, weddings, birthdays, or holidays. You could even rightfully argue that it's inappropriate not to participate in special family and social events and the food that goes with them.

On the other hand, bingeing alone at home after a stressful event is an inappropriate use of food for nonphysical reasons. When I surveyed my coaching group members recently, every one of them told me they had used eating or drinking sometime in the past six months to cope with stress or depression. The irony is that emotional hunger can never be satisfied with food.

Lisa, one of my personal clients from New Jersey, was over two hundred pounds when she first came to see me. What struck me at first was how much she knew about training and nutrition. The problem, in her own words, was that she couldn't stop eating. Giving her my standard lecture about what to eat would have been pointless. Instead, we explored the reasons why she was overeating and discovered that she ate to feel better when she was alone or depressed. Food doesn't solve these problems.

We did two simple things: first, we identified the right reasons to eat—for fuel, nutrition, health, and building muscle—and we programmed that into her mind using affirmations and the mental training tools you'll learn about in the next chapter. Second, we found alternative ways for her to get the good feelings she was after. We brainstormed how she could become more socially active, inside and outside the gym, and we listed things she could do instead of eating when she was feeling down.

Lisa did not go on a new diet, she installed new ideas in her mind. It was a massive breakthrough and her results were beyond our expectations. She dropped thirty-two pounds in the next twelve weeks. Today she is a personal trainer and a great role model for her clients.

The solution begins with awareness. Once you're consciously aware of the reasons you eat, you can catch yourself before eating emotionally. At those important moments of decision, you can reframe the situation and tell yourself, "I'm not hungry, I'm just feeling upset." When you consciously realize that food is only a quick fix for feeling better, you can use alternative coping mechanisms or substitute more appropriate behaviors to satisfy the feeling.

According to research by Dr. Brian Wansink, author of *Mindless Eating*, you make as many as two hundred decisions about food every day, ranging from what to have for breakfast, to whether to eat every time you pass a candy dish. If you make your decisions about food emotionally, the impact on your weight and health can be very destructive over time.

To catch yourself from making impulsive decisions, a good first step is to fine-tune your senses to recognize the difference between real hunger and emotional hunger. You also need to recognize the difference between a slight physical hunger, which sometimes must be tolerated, and a sharp physical hunger, indicating a real need for fuel.

How to Tell the Difference
Between Physical and Emotional Hunger

There are some very distinct differences between physical and emotional hunger.

- Physical hunger builds up gradually, starting with a tiny grumble in the stomach, growing to full-blown hunger pangs. Emotional hunger develops suddenly.
- With physical hunger, you can wait if you have to. Emotional hunger seems to demand immediate satisfaction.

- Physical hunger usually appears about three hours after the last meal or snack. Emotional hunger can happen anytime.
- Physical hunger is usually a general desire for food. Emotional hunger is usually a desire for a specific food.
- After eating for physical hunger, the hunger goes away. After emotional eating, the hunger persists.
- After eating for physical hunger, you get a sense of satisfaction. After eating for emotional reasons, you feel guilty.

The Truth About Physical Hunger and Dietary Restraint

Many dietitians and psychologists teach that you should eat when you're hungry. If their intention is that you need to eat in response to real physical hunger, not emotional hunger, then I agree. However, if you interpret this literally as, "Always eat every time you're physically hungry," then I don't believe it's good advice. What if you've already met your caloric allowance for the day but you're still physically hungry?

If you want to get leaner, you must establish a caloric deficit, which means you're probably going to be hungry sometimes. If you respond to every slight sensation of physical hunger as a signal to eat, you may be canceling your caloric deficit. I'm not talking about starvation diets that create ravenous hunger. I'm talking about maintaining a small caloric deficit, tolerating a little bit of occasional hunger and having some dietary restraint.

It's impossible to ignore the type of true physical hunger that's experienced under starvation conditions because hunger is the most primal human drive—even more primal than reproduction. Landmark research on starvation performed by Ancel Keys at the University of Minnesota many years ago revealed that when subjects were fed a semistarvation diet at 50 percent of their maintenance caloric intake for six months, the drive to eat became obsessive and all-encompassing. The subjects could not think of anything but food. They even lost interest in sex.

This makes complete sense from a survival point of view because if you were starving and couldn't feed yourself, you'd be in no condition to bear and feed offspring. During starvation, appetite hormones automatically increase while sex drive and reproductive functions decrease. On low-calorie diets and at extremely low body-fat levels, women's menstrual cycles stop and men's testosterone levels plummet.

This makes a good case for avoiding extreme low-calorie diets because you can never fight the primal hunger urge forever. It's a lot like sleep. You can deprive yourself for a while, at great cost to your well-being, but ultimately you can't resist the urge. On the other hand, anyone who tells you that achieving and maintaining your ideal weight doesn't require any dietary restraint is being unrealistic. You must become aware of your body's signals and learn to respond appropriately to them. That might mean not eating more, even if you feel like it.

A great example of dietary restraint can be seen among the Okinawans, who are among the leanest and longest-lived populations in the world. The Okinawan culture has a tradition known as *hari hachi bu*, which means, "Eat until you're only 80 percent full." Contrast that with the Western cultural practice of "cleaning your plate" and "not wasting food" and we may have one answer to why there's an obesity crisis in America today.

Stop "Waisting" Your Food

Through years of social conditioning from your parents and culture, you may have developed a belief that you must clean all the food off your plate, whether you're still hungry or not. You may have been programmed to believe that it's insulting to your host not to eat everything you're served, that it's throwing away money if you don't eat everything you paid for, or that you shouldn't waste food when there are less fortunate people in the world who are starving.

May I suggest a different perspective? If you continue eating after you're already full, then you're wasting food anyway because fullness is a fairly dependable signal that your energy needs are already met. You don't need that much caloric energy, so the excess gets stored as adipose tissue . . . and that's a real "waist." By the way, if you can prove to me that clearing everything off your plate will help starving children in Africa, let me know exactly how it helps and then I'll join you.

Remember that one of the essential success beliefs of lean people is willingness. We don't do "wishful thinking" in the Body Fat Solution program, we do accurate thinking and we become willing to do whatever it takes. A little bit of hunger should be expected while you're in a calorie deficit and it's part of the price you pay for getting leaner.

The real issue is, how do you most effectively deal with the hunger? Cognitive psychologist Judith Beck, Ph.D., provides some excellent advice on tolerating hunger in her book *The Beck Diet Solution*:

> **YOU DEFINITELY DON'T HAVE TO EAT** when you're hungry. Just because you want to eat doesn't mean you always should. If you fear hunger, you might routinely eat to avoid the feeling. You can learn to tolerate hunger. Remind yourself that there have been times in your life when you've been hungry and survived. You'll always survive because hunger is never an emergency.

Another way to handle hunger is to use your new reframing skills. If a caloric deficit causes fat cells to shrink and if a little bit of hunger comes with a calorie deficit, then why not change your perspective: "It's not hunger, it's the feeling of fat cells shrinking!"

The A.W.A.R.E. Formula: Five Steps That End Emotional Eating

Awareness is the starting point of change, because you can't solve a problem if you don't know you have one. You're about to learn how to develop a keen awareness of your behavior patterns, how to stop negative patterns dead in their tracks, and how to replace them with positive new ones. You'll also learn how to make the changes permanent by literally rewiring your nervous system so the negative patterns are less likely to occur and positive new eating behaviors will run on autopilot.

There are five simple steps to this process, which I call the A.W.A.R.E. formula:

1. Become AWARE of your eating behaviors.
2. WATCH OUT for your emotional eating triggers.
3. ARREST the behavior patterns when they happen.
4. REPLACE the old emotional eating behavior with more constructive alternatives.
5. ESTABLISH new beliefs about food and the right reasons for eating.

Let's take a closer look at each of the five steps.

STEP 1: Become AWARE of Your Eating Behaviors

At first, your biggest challenge is that you don't even realize when you're eating emotionally. In a word, you eat "mindlessly." We all use free will and make conscious decisions, but 95 percent of our daily behaviors run on automatic pilot. These unconsciously driven behaviors are known as habits.

You don't have to think about beating your heart, releasing hormones, or digesting your food because these are autopilot bodily functions handled by your autonomic nervous system. If your unconscious mind has the power to handle such enormous and complex physiological tasks, then you can understand how easily it can also create and carry out automatic eating behaviors without consulting your conscious mind.

For example, if stress eating has become an unconscious pattern, you don't have to think about what to do when you feel stressed. A line of code has been installed in your brain that says, "If there's stress, then eat comfort food."

You eat without thinking for many reasons, and the neural associations to foods that trigger emotional eating can be formed at a very young age. Foods can get linked to home, family, friends, love, being pampered, and just about any person, place, or experience.

On my new-client work sheet are two questions whose answers I always look at very closely. The first is, "What are your favorite foods?" The second is, "Why are those your favorite foods?" Sometimes my clients give superficial answers such as, "I like the taste." But when I ask more questions, I usually find a memory associated with every favorite food. When I probe deep enough, I hear answers like, "That flavor of ice cream reminds me of summers at the beach house when I was a kid. Those were good times." In this case, ice cream had been linked to all the emotions related to family, summer fun, and the carefree days of childhood. Those days may be long gone, but the ice cream is always there as a way to recapture the feelings.

Since habitual eating patterns can go back so far and they're programmed at the unconscious level, they'll continue to run on automatic pilot unless you intentionally break them and replace them with new ones. However, before you can break an old pattern, you must know it exists. That's where awareness comes in. You must start paying attention. Some people call this conscious or mindful eating and it's the polar opposite of mindless or impulse eating.

There are two important aspects to eating with awareness. The first is eating exclusively, which means that when you eat, you do nothing but eat. Studies show that TV viewing time correlates highly with weight gain, obesity, and weight regain. One explanation is that while watching TV, it's easy to get a surplus of calories because while you're occupied with what's on the TV screen, you don't pay attention to how much you're consuming.

Eating exclusively also helps prevent you from forming undesirable neural associations through stimulus-response conditioning, also known as the "Pavlov's dog effect." Watching TV, reading the newspaper, working on your computer, or any other stimulus can become linked to eating if you pair the two activities together often enough. If the TV becomes anchored to eating, then even if you're not physically hungry, just sitting in front of the TV will neurologically trigger the thought of eating.

The second aspect of mindful eating is to eat slowly. "Don't inhale your food" isn't just an admonishment that you probably heard from your mother, it's scientifically accurate weight control advice. The effect of eating slowly, which scientists call "time-energy displacement," has been studied extensively. Eating too quickly doesn't allow the satiety mechanisms in your brain to register the caloric energy. By the time you feel full, you may have already eaten too much.

A recent study at the University of Alabama discovered something that might be more important than eating slowly. After looking at satiety (how full a food makes you feel), energy density (calories per unit of volume), and eating time of various foods, researchers found it was even more advantageous to choose foods that *force* you to ingest calories more slowly, so you couldn't consume the calories faster if you tried.

This means choosing foods with a high satiety factor, a high "chew factor," and a low energy density (such as high-fiber vegetables and lean proteins), and fewer foods with a low satiety factor and a high energy density (such as liquid calories, refined sugars, and grains). You'll learn more about this high-low approach to fat-burning nutrition in Chapter Six.

Another way to raise conscious awareness is to keep a journal, including a daily record of your nutritional intake, as well as a diary of your thoughts and feelings before, during, and after you eat. I recommend journaling for at least four to twelve weeks when you first start the program and again at any time you want to work on an important goal or if you think you're slipping back. Continuing to keep a food journal into the maintenance phase is your choice, but in the early stages when you're developing new habits, journaling provides a learning experience and awareness exercise that's unequaled any other way.

A journal can be a real wake-up call as you begin to realize the extent of your old emotional and impulse eating behaviors. As your journal makes you accountable for what, when, how much, and why you've been eating, you may notice some of your behaviors start to change and your results improve instantly, just because you're keeping track.

STEP 2: WATCH OUT for Your Emotional Eating Triggers

Emotional eating doesn't happen without a reason. There's always a cause. We all have numerous triggers or cues, and the more of them you can identify, the better. During the initial period when you're breaking old habit patterns and establishing new ones, think of your conscious mind as the police. If you know in advance where the "scene of the crime" will be, then you can stake out the scene, be on guard, and arrest the old negative pattern before it's carried out.

So it's time for a little detective work. What pushes your emotional eating buttons? Check off anything that applies to you and add anything else you can think of that's not on the list. As you make your own list, keep in mind that triggers generally fall into one of four categories; feelings, places, people, or events. Some triggers are under your control, others are not.

- stress
- loneliness
- boredom
- anger
- frustration
- sadness
- feeling ignored
- feeling unloved
- feeling worthless
- overwork
- overwhelm
- fatigue or exhaustion
- financial challenges
- relationship challenges
- parties
- holidays
- weather

- buffets
- restaurants
- food in the kitchen
- food in the office
- the refrigerator
- smell of food
- sight of food
- people offering you food
- people eating food around you
- time of day
- time of month
- television
- going to the movies
- your mom's cooking
- your spouse's cooking
- other: _____

Once you've identified your triggers, your goal is to remove the ones you control and prepare your defenses for those you don't. Doing a clean sweep of your home and office is good place to start because easy access to snack foods is a major trigger for most people. Convenience leads to mindless eating. If it's not there, you can't eat it. If possible, get the convenience foods out of your house and office. At the very least, keep them out of reach and out of sight.

If your primary triggers are people, then you can create social coping strategies in advance. First, tell your friends and family what you're doing and ask them to support you unconditionally. If there are any situations or relationships where you still anticipate peer pressure or invitations to eat too much food or the wrong foods, plan a rebuttal for every comment you're likely to hear. The reframing skills you learned in Chapter Three will come in handy. Here are some ideas:

- Maybe it does taste good, but nothing tastes as good as being lean feels.
- It's not about missing out on sweets, it's about missing out on being a lean person.
- It's not about losing freedom to eat what I want, it's about not being a slave to food.
- It's not about eating with family, it's about being with family.

Stress as an Emotional Eating Trigger

One of the most common triggers for emotional eating is stress. One of the simplest ways to handle stress is to change the way you perceive it. Stress is not inherently problematic. What matters most is how you interpret and respond to it. What if you changed some of your beliefs and reframed your experience of stress, like this:

- Stress is an essential part of life because stress is the stimulus for growth.
- Stress is okay. What's bad for me is continuous stress without release. When I feel constant stress is starting to pressure me, that's my signal to rest, relax, and recover. I work hard and sometimes it's stressful, but then I play hard and recover.
- It's not food that I really want or need when I feel overstressed, it's rest and relaxation. Feeling stressed simply means I need a better balance between stress and relaxation.

- Use food when I feel stressed? No way! Food is good for energy and nutrition, but it's a terrible way to de-stress because stress eating only makes me feel guilty afterward, and guilt means even more stress.

STEP 3: ARREST the Negative Patterns When They Happen

As your level of awareness increases, you'll change from an unconscious eater to a conscious eater. This gives you the opportunity to interrupt or arrest the negative pattern before carrying it out. I like the concept of arresting negative patterns because it implies that you've been "policing" your thoughts, feelings, environment, and behaviors so you can catch yourself in the act.

When you become aware of an urge to eat inappropriately, it's an important moment of decision. Awareness gives you the chance to have a conversation with yourself in those critical moments before you act. Start by simply saying, "Stop!" or "Wait!" Then apply some "creative procrastination." Remind yourself, "I could always eat this later, but for now, let me think about what eating this might do to me."

The important thing is to stop, pause, and think before you eat. That gives you time to ask yourself some important questions:

- Am I thinking about eating because I'm physically hungry or for another reason?
- If it's not for physical hunger, then why am I thinking about eating this?
- What will be the immediate consequences if I eat this?
- What will be the long-term consequences if I eat this?
- What will be my rewards for saying no to this?
- Is eating this going to move me closer to or farther away from my goal?
- Is eating this worth it?

When you're asking yourself about the consequences, it helps to see with long-term perspective and project the potential consequences far into the future. Personally, I find the concept of "I am what I eat" arrests the pattern quite well.

I ask myself, "Do I really want to eat this processed, unnatural food if it's going to become a part of every cell in my body—my muscles, my brain, my lungs, or even my eyeballs?"

Then I ask myself, "How will I feel after I've eaten this?" This one is usually the reality check. The illusion is that food will make you feel better. The reality is that you'll feel worse after eating to feed emotional hunger. You'll feel better after eating for the right reasons and finding more constructive ways to cope with your feelings.

STEP 4: REPLACE the Old Emotional Eating Behavior with More Constructive Alternatives

There are always constructive ways to obtain or satisfy any feeling. It's not about the food, it's about getting the feeling you thought you'd get from eating that food. What are you really hungry for? Companionship? Love? Happiness? If you could get the same feelings in some way other than eating, then why don't you? What if you found out that eating that food provided only short-term pleasure followed by long-term pain? Would you still eat it?

All of my coaching protégés who have successfully overcome emotional eating have two things in common. First, they realized that eating inappropriately would make them feel worse, not better. Tanya, for example, was a thirty-six-year-old single entrepreneur. She told me she had begun to gain weight in her thirties, and she believed it was from stress and lack of time for exercise. The turning point for her was the moment she realized that her eating for stress relief didn't relieve anything; it actually created more stress through guilt:

> **I USED TO BELIEVE** that eating would make me feel good, but now I realize that overeating only made me feel sluggish, bloated, and guilty afterward. It wasn't worth it for any short-lived relief I got. What really makes me feel good is being in control and the victory I feel from becoming fitter, healthier, and better than I was yesterday.

The second trait I found in everyone who overcame stress eating was the ability to develop alternate coping mechanisms.

Some people, when they become depressed, drown their sorrows in alcohol or engage in episodes of binge eating. Others seek professional help or call their closest friends and loved ones and talk their way through it. Social support and a sympathetic pair of ears can be powerfully therapeutic.

Some people reach for food when they feel stressed. Other people find ways to relax: they take up meditation or yoga, light candles, play relaxing music, take a hot bath, soak in the Jacuzzi, do some deep breathing exercises, or go for a slow walk down the beach or through the woods. Some people simply remove themselves from the source of the stress and take time off, if possible.

Some people come home from work fatigued or exhausted and immediately reach for food. Other people take a power nap and then focus on improving the quality of their nighttime sleep.

Some people reach for food when they're upset or angry. Other people "work it out." They hit the gym, go for a run, punch a heavy bag, or take a kick-boxing class.

When you feel the temptation to feed emotional hunger, distracting yourself by doing some kind of physical activity like walking can be a helpful strategy. The benefits of physical activity, however, go far beyond mere distraction. Physical movement and exercise might be the single best way to change how you feel because your mind and body are connected. Emotion follows motion. When you move your body, you change the way you feel. The worst thing you can do is nothing.

STEP 5: ESTABLISH New Beliefs About Food and the Right Reasons for Eating

One of the most powerful strategies for ending emotional eating or any other undesirable eating habit is one that few people consider: examine your beliefs about food and what food means to you and, if necessary, change them.

What is it that makes certain eating behaviors possible for some people but unthinkable for others? It's not that some people have superhuman willpower that lets them easily say no to every temptation. When a behavior violates your strongest beliefs, there is no temptation. For example, what keeps a vegetarian from eating meat? If she has spiritual and humanitarian reasons for her choice and she's fully aware of those reasons, then it's not hard to avoid meat; eating meat would feel totally incongruent, maybe even repulsive.

Most people are totally unaware of their beliefs about food and how they affect their behaviors and decisions. A surefire way to know a person's beliefs is by looking at their results. As the proverb goes, "By their fruits you shall know them." You can also uncover a person's beliefs by listening closely to their language.

Beliefs and the Power of Metaphor

In many of the mind-body healing disciplines, it's believed that people express what's going on in their bodies in the form of body talk, also known as somatic metaphors, for example, "pain in the neck," "It makes my blood boil," "I don't want to hear it," and so on. Whether or not you believe that a somatic metaphor could actually cause a disease (psychosomatic illness) is up to you.

I believe that metaphor is a language the unconscious mind can understand, so by changing the metaphors you use to describe your body and the food you eat, you can help initiate a change in your belief systems and subsequently your behaviors.

If you believed your body was a temple or a divine gift, would you desecrate it by poisoning it with junk food? What if you said your body was like a high-performance sports car? Do you think you might fuel it differently? If you believed your body was a lean, fat-burning machine, how do you think it might affect your attitude toward training? How would it change your response to adversity if you described yourself as a warrior? Most people don't realize that innocent labels and nicknames can actually change behavior and mold an identity. If you're going to label yourself anyway, why not choose empowering labels?

When it comes to food, I've discovered that fit, lean, and healthy people have a unique set of beliefs about food and a distinct set of metaphors they use to describe food and what food is for. The ones I've heard most often include:

- Food is fuel.
- Food is the best medicine.
- Food is construction material for the body.
- Food stokes the fire of metabolism.
- Fruit is nature's candy.
- Lean protein is the lean muscle builder.
- High-fiber foods are nature's Roto-Rooter.

I've never met anyone who talked about food with this type of language exclusively, who had a challenge with inappropriate eating or excess body fat. Think about that. When you look at it this way, food is no longer the problem, food is the solution and you become driven to eat the right foods rather than avoid food.

If you use metaphors to describe the food you eat, write them all down so you become more aware of them. Discard the negative ones and keep the positive ones. If you don't use any yet, make a list of all the metaphors you could start using today that would influence your attitudes, beliefs, and behaviors in a positive way.

Identifying and Replacing Beliefs About Food That Lead to Emotional Eating

Let me emphasize again just how important this fifth step of belief change really is, because awareness alone is not enough. It's one thing to raise your awareness, but you can become conscious of destructive emotional eating behaviors and still feel powerless to stop them. Where the real change takes place is in your beliefs, because your beliefs and other unconscious programs are the core drivers of your behavior.

If you want to change a behavior, you need to change the beliefs that mobilize the behavior. Your task is to uncover your beliefs about diet, nutrition, and food and bring them into conscious awareness. This requires a little bit of brainstorming, and you should take your time and list as many of your food beliefs as you can think of.

Dan, one of my coaching clients, came up with this list:

- Breakfast is the most important meal of the day.
- Food is for energy.
- I deserve a good cheat meal on the weekends if I had a good week.
- It's important to avoid artificial chemicals.
- It's good to eat as organic as possible.
- High protein is important for building muscle.
- It's impossible to eat the right foods when I'm traveling a lot.

After you have your beliefs on paper, then separate them into two categories: empowering and limiting. Ask yourself, "Does believing this move me toward my goal or away from it?"

When I read Dan's list, I saw that most of his beliefs about food were arguably helpful, but I asked him if he thought any of them were holding him back. It was no surprise which one he picked out.

When you identify the beliefs about food that aren't serving you, you can use the reframing and belief change techniques you learned in Chapter Three to replace them. In Dan's case, we found a single belief that it was "impossible" to eat right while traveling created a major bottleneck in his progress.

When I suggested that he could come home from every trip in better shape than when he left, it completely "scrambled his brain" at first because it didn't fit with his current paradigm. It wasn't difficult to change his mind, however. I showed him how other people had done it, we focused his attention on pretrip planning and preparation, and then I made a huge list of travel eating and training strategies. In the end, Dan became positively obsessed with the idea of getting in better shape every time he traveled. He actually replaced his old limiting belief about food with its polar opposite. Within months, he was in the best shape of his life.

Remember, replacement is the key, not removal, so always choose and write down the empowering new beliefs you want to put in place of the old ones. In the next chapter, you'll learn more about how to write affirmations, set goals, and use mental training to plant these new beliefs in your unconscious mind so they'll become your new pattern that plays on autopilot in the future.

Four Core Beliefs That Highly Fit and Lean People Have About Food

I consider a person's beliefs about health to be sacred, so I'm not going to suggest that you take on any specific beliefs unless you feel comfortable doing so. However, there are several key beliefs about food that I've found to be extremely valuable to help develop the type of relationship with food that optimizes health and fitness. Following are the four beliefs and an affirmation for each one.

1. Food is for building material

"Food is construction material for the body. I will become what I eat, as food literally becomes the cells, organs, and tissues of my body."

2. Food is for fuel

"Food is fuel. I will be as energetic as the fuel I put into my bodily engine."

3. Food is for nourishment

"Nutritious foods contain everything I need for perfect health."

4. Food is for stoking the metabolic fire

"When I feed myself nourishing food on a consistent meal schedule, it stokes my metabolic furnace."

I've discovered that nearly all highly fit and lean people hold these or similar beliefs. "Food is fuel," for example, is a very powerful and important belief for a fitness-seeking person to possess. I don't remember ever meeting a highly fit and lean person who didn't believe this.

Adopting these types of beliefs could transform your relationship with food. These are also unemotional beliefs about food. They're essentially saying, "It's just food." They strip away the intense feelings we tend to associate with food. As you begin to adopt, affirm, and imprint these beliefs into your nervous system, food begins to lose its emotional pull over you and you start to feel compelled to eat the right foods for the right reasons.

There is a catch, however, to de-emotionalizing your relationship with food. If you lived your life only believing these four things about food, you might easily develop the physique of an athlete or fitness model. But without having some other beliefs that ensure balance and long-term happiness, you might be depriving yourself of the appropriate use of one of life's great enjoyments and the social rewards that go along with it.

Ten Beliefs and Affirmations About Food for Balance, Happiness, and Long-term Success

1. "It's okay to eat for enjoyment or social reasons if I do it consciously and mindfully and I stay within the compliance rules and quantity limits I set for myself in advance."
2. "I'm totally conscious and aware of my beliefs about food and the reasons I eat."

3. "When I feel stressed or depressed, I have alternate ways to cope with those feelings."

4. "Healthy food that helps me burn fat and build muscle can be prepared in delicious ways."

5. "I realize that food can be one of life's great pleasures and that completely denying myself of foods I enjoy is not productive in the long run."

6. "I don't have to be perfect. If I eat healthy, natural foods at least 90 percent of the time, I know I will get good results."

7. "If I set a compliance rule for myself, then there's no such thing as forbidden foods. As long as I obey the law of calorie balance and eat only small amounts, I can still be healthy, develop a great body, *and* enjoy my favorite foods in moderation."

8. "If I want better results, faster, I realize that I may need to tighten up my nutritional compliance and I'm willing to do it if that's what it takes."

9. "Everything I eat will have some effect on my body, but I realize that what I eat once in a while doesn't impact me that much."

10. "What's most important is what I eat habitually, so I'm very conscious about what I eat repeatedly day after day. I understand and have great respect for the power of habits."

The Importance of Appropriate Behavior

Some goals take extreme physical effort, mental strength, and discipline, along with a different and unique set of beliefs and much higher standards. But you would probably live a lonely and isolated life of denial if you were nothing but an emotionless robot, feeding "the machine" for nothing but fuel and growth, 100 percent of the time.

You can achieve a healthy balance in life more easily when you understand and practice appropriate behavior. If you struggle with your weight, it's not because you eat ice cream once in a while with your kids or you want a piece of decadent double chocolate cake when dining out at a nice restaurant on a special occasion. That's perfectly normal. Your troubles begin when you use ice cream and other comfort foods inappropriately as a coping mechanism, especially if you do it mindlessly and frequently.

Give yourself permission to enjoy foods that are outside your usual eating rules, provided you enjoy them appropriately, which means infrequently for special occasions and in a restrained manner. By doing so, you'll develop an exquisite balance between the health and fitness side of your life and the social and recreational side and you'll never struggle with food again.

Belief Power Versus Willpower—No Contest

Without question, the most powerful ways to end emotional eating are by increasing your awareness and establishing a belief system that short-circuits eating for the wrong reasons while triggering eating for the right reasons. Belief power is a thousand times stronger than willpower because belief power uses the unconscious mind to create behavior change with automation, while willpower uses the conscious mind to create behavior change with force.

Once you harness the power of belief and all the other strategies you've learned in this and the previous three chapters, it won't be long before eating for the right reasons will become your new unconscious programming. Eventually, it will become a part of who you are. You are a lean healthy person, or in the process of becoming one.

Only one-third of the way through this book, you now understand the root causes of body fat, you've learned the truth about common body fat myths, you've gained new perspectives, installed new beliefs, and you have all the tools you need to end emotional eating. This means that the stage has been set, your mind has been prepared, and you're ready to begin learning some real-world action strategies. When you combine all these mental and emotional tools with the proven nutrition and training strategies you're about to learn in part two, you will have a combination that virtually guarantees your success.

PART TWO

THE FIVE PRINCIPLES

Mental Training Solution

Setting Goals and Reprogramming Your Mind for Automatic Success

> DISCOVERIES in the science of cybernetics point to the conclusion that your brain and nervous system constitute a goal-striving mechanism which operates automatically to achieve your goal, very much as a self-aiming torpedo or missile seeks out its target and steers its way to it.
>
> —DR. MAXWELL MALTZ, AUTHOR OF *PSYCHO-CYBERNETICS*

In 1967, Dr. Charles Garfield took a position as a mathematician on the Apollo 11 moon project. He was surrounded every day by some of the world's highest achievers, and began to realize that individuals who excelled at their profession shared certain unique characteristics. This started an intensive journey that led him to study the world's greatest athletes and business successes.

After sixteen years and more than fifteen hundred interviews, he isolated the specific qualities that enabled top achievers to excel in their fields. He published his findings in his 1984 book, *Peak Performance: Mental Training Techniques of the World's Greatest Athletes*. Garfield discovered that the secret to high performance in sports was the same in business, science, arts, and academics. It's also the same secret that unlocks success in personal fitness and weight management.

Garfield's discovery was also influenced by the outcome of the 1976 Olympics, where the Russians and East Germans so completely dominated the competition that accusations of steroid use were flying. Toward the end of 1976, information leaked out that the Eastern bloc athletes had been using "mental training sessions." It didn't take long before coaches and psychologists in the West were pursuing research of their own to investigate this Soviet "secret weapon."

Both medical and psychological research began to uncover astounding ways in which the mind and emotions could affect the body. Blood flow, nutrient absorption, transfer of oxygen, and even hormonal activity could all be affected by mental state. Pregame excitement could affect the autonomic nervous system and improve performance. Negative emotions such as worry, self-doubt, and anxiety could also influence the body and cause detrimental effects on performance.

Most interesting of all, athletes who engaged in mental training reported a peak state that later became known as "flow." Distractions fell into the background, awareness was heightened, focus sharpened, and the athlete was filled with a sense of power and expectation of success.

While in this peak state, some athletes said they felt as though they were acting automatically. The winning quarterback would throw the ball to the right place at just the right moment without a second of conscious deliberation. World-champion boxers swore that their fists seemed to take on a mind of their own, striking without being commanded to do so. It was as if the athletes were released from conscious thought during those critical moments and something else took over. As it turns out, that's *exactly* what happened.

Nearly a decade earlier, a plastic surgeon named Maxwell Maltz had already been teaching millions of people about the power of the unconscious mind to change behavior, achieve goals, increase self-confidence, and alter the self-image. In his 1960 book *Psycho-Cybernetics*, which still sells today, Maltz explained that the unconscious was capable of guiding flawless execution of sports skills at critical high-pressure moments. It was also the part of the mind responsible for automation of behavior patterns that we commonly call habits.

The unconscious was formally discussed in a scientific fashion as early as the sixteenth century. Near the turn of the twentieth century, Sigmund Freud made the first clear, albeit crude, distinction of the unconscious as a force that drove human behavior. It was Maltz, however, who made a real breakthrough, with two profound discoveries.

Your Brain: Goal-Seeking Supercomputer

First, he recognized that the unconscious was a goal-seeking mechanism that could not be turned off. Second, he said that the mind was like a computer and could be programmed or reprogrammed. Together, Maltz said these characteristics allowed the human mind to work like a guidance system, similar to the way a torpedo or missile homes in on its target. Once locked on a target, the "servo-mechanism" would recognize if you drifted off course and guide you back to your target. This type of self-correcting mechanism is known as cybernetic, from the Greek word for "steersman."

Suppose you were entrusted with the job of torpedo launcher and your mission was to enter the coordinates of the target into the torpedo's onboard guidance system. What would happen if you launched the torpedo into the ocean without programming any target into the onboard computer? Without a target, the torpedo would go around in circles or hit something unintended. If there was no propulsion, it would just sink.

Firing a torpedo with no target would be ludicrous, but that's exactly what you're doing every day if you don't program your mind with goals. Goals are your personal life targets, and that includes your ideal body and ideal weight. To reach your goals, there are two necessary steps. First you must choose a target and second, as Garfield emphasized, you must program that target into your mental computer:

> **THE FOUNDATION** of every peak performer's training is contained in a single word: program. I would like to emblazon this word on a billboard in letters nine feet tall to emphasize this point. Without the structure provided by a clear, step-by-step training program, the athlete can waste precious hours, or even years, seeking a path to excellence down cul-de-sacs where little or nothing is accomplished.

The Real Secret to All Success

Many psychologists claim that most of our programming is planted in our unconscious minds at a very young age and can't be changed. They're only right about the first part. You have all kinds of programming in your mind put there by parents, teachers, friends, media, and culture. A lot of it was unhelpful. A lot of it is still there. Fortunately, you can reprogram your mind with new targets and change the direction of your life at any age.

One problem is, you didn't get a user's manual for the brain when you were born, and they don't teach this stuff in school. Another problem is that even though more thought leaders than ever are now teaching how to use your brain for behavior change and personal achievement, much of the information is delivered in a mystical or pseudoscientific package. This contributes to skepticism and adds to the number of critics who say it's all a bunch of baloney.

You need only look at Olympic and professional sports to see that mental training is serious business. Today, advances in neuroscience and brain imaging technologies such as functional MRI, PET, and SPECT scans have continued to validate the effectiveness of mental training. The real secret of success is to understand and intentionally use the power of your unconscious mind. It's the key to the body of your dreams and everything else you want in life.

You Think Less Than You Think

Did you ever do something completely illogical or totally opposite of what you said you wanted? Afterward, did you say to yourself, "Why did I do that?" Why would you scarf down an entire bag of cookies in a binge when your conscious desire is to get a leaner and healthier body? Why would you skip a workout when your conscious desire is to become fitter, stronger, and more muscular?

You have the free will to consciously choose any action and make any decision. Most people, however, are totally unaware of the degree of "automaticity" at work in their daily lives. Research by Dr. John Bargh of Yale University suggests that up to 95 percent of your behavior is unconsciously chosen. Some experts believe the unconscious makes up as much as 99 percent of your brain's functions and that conscious thinking is nothing but the tip of a massive iceberg. An enormous amount of mental activity is going on below the level of your conscious awareness.

It seems like you're willfully choosing every action because you notice a thought pop into your head before you do something. You say to yourself, "I'm going to the gym," and then you go to the gym. You say, "I want some ice cream," and then you go get some ice cream. However, even when you think about something before you do it, that conscious thought may have bubbled up from the unconscious level.

Your Brain Works Faster Than You Can Think

Not only does most of your mental activity take place on the unconscious level, but the unconscious processing also happens faster than your conscious mind can think. Research on subliminal perception has shown that you can't consciously see a picture that's flashed on a screen for less than fifty milliseconds, but your nonconscious neurons can perceive it.

Electrical impulses in your brain can fire in milliseconds, allowing you to react to stimuli that you haven't consciously noticed. This is helpful to the elite athlete who must perform complex skills with precision. It also helps in everyday situations where you must make split-second judgments or act quickly to keep you out of harm's way.

Unfortunately, this may also explain why you do things impulsively, such as overeat or skip workouts. Research by William Gehring and Adrian Willoughby from the University of Michigan found that unconscious processing occurs so fast that impulsive decisions can be made without consulting your conscious mind.

Turning Positive Behaviors to "Autopilot" Mode

Some body functions, such as breathing, can be consciously controlled, but you don't need to think about circulating your blood, releasing hormones, digesting your food, healing cuts, or creating new cells. That's a good thing because the complexity of all your bodily systems is more than the conscious mind can handle. Your unconscious mind is the command center that handles autonomic body functions. It also controls automatic behaviors and can easily turn any behavior over to autopilot mode.

Driving a car, for example, is a very unconscious activity, even though conscious attention is required. Do you remember how complicated it seemed the first time you tried to drive, especially a stick shift? At first it seemed like there were a dozen things demanding your attention at once, but after a while it became so second nature, you hardly had to think at all. In fact, you can probably recall occasions when you slipped into a "driving trance" and didn't remember the last few miles you traveled. Who was driving the car then?

What if you could put productive eating and exercise behaviors on autopilot? Well, you can. Your unconscious mind excels at taking over routine tasks and helping you do them automatically or very easily with little conscious thought. Anything can get turned over to habit with enough practice or repetition. This prevents your conscious mind from being overloaded and allows you to concentrate your precious conscious resources on more important things.

The Reticular Activating System— Your Brain's "Important List"

The retinas of your eyes can process up to ten million bits of data per second. You take in another one million bits through your other senses. Your conscious mind, however, can only process about forty bits per second. That's the average speed of information processing while reading. The amount of data your conscious mind can hold is very limited. Cognitive psychologist George Miller set the magic number at chunks of seven plus or minus two. Coincidentally, seven is the number of digits in a phone number.

One of the ways your brain handles the information overload is by deleting things it evaluates as unimportant. The part of your brain responsible for this is called the reticular activating system (RAS). All the data that comes into your brain through your eyes and other senses is filtered through the RAS.

One of the functions of the RAS is to decide whether something should be called to your conscious attention or get filed away in the unconscious parts of the brain for future use. This is why some scientists call the RAS the attention center, or "important list," in your brain. If impulses are sent to your conscious mind, you'll notice them and usually respond to them immediately.

Attention, Attraction, and the Unconscious Mind in Goal Achievement

Let's suppose you want a new car—a blue BMW Z4. It starts off as nothing but an idea in your head, but once you decide, you start thinking about that car all the time. That's how the achievement of any goal begins. When you think about something a lot, and especially when you write it down and stay focused on it, you're telling your brain that it's important to you. All of a sudden, your brain brings to your attention everything in your environment that has any relevance to getting your goal.

You start to notice the auto magazines on the newsstand, as well as TV commercials, classified ads in the newspaper, Web pages that talk about

BMWs, dealerships when you pass by, you hear someone all the way across the room talking about BMWs, and all of sudden you see blue BMWs on the road everywhere. Well, guess what? Those BMWs were on the road already, people were already talking about BMWs, magazine articles and ads were already written about BMWs, you simply didn't notice them. Why? Because your brain didn't think it was important and filtered it out of your conscious awareness.

This attention mechanism in your mind is so powerful, it starts to seem as if everything you need to get your goal is being "attracted" to you or that things are happening through "mystical coincidences." What's really happening is your brain is making you notice things you didn't notice before. Most scientists don't accept that "attraction" is a physical law of the universe. But it's certainly an observable psychological phenomenon and you'll learn in Chapter Nine that it's also a very real social phenomenon, ("Birds of a feather flock together").

Setting a goal shifts your brain's perception and attention, therefore attracting what you want from the outside in. Setting goals also causes changes from the inside out. When you get a goal on your important list, your brain searches its memory banks for anything you've ever read, heard, or experienced having anything to do with your goal. Great ideas for reaching your goal seem to pop up inside your head. Hunches, intuitions, and gut feelings do not come from "out there," they bubble up from inside your mind.

Then, your behavior starts to change automatically. You might get the sudden urge to put in overtime to earn more money. If you're in sales, your closing ratio improves and you earn higher commissions. You start working harder to get a raise, bonus, or promotion. You invest more carefully. You cut back on expenses and save money. You might get the motivation to start a new part-time business.

The goal achievement process begins with nothing but an idea in your head—"I want X." When X becomes your dominating thought, it goes high on your important list, your attention shifts, and your behavior changes. The new-car phenomenon is the most commonly quoted example of the RAS and unconscious mind in action, but think about the astounding implications of this for achieving all your goals in life, including your ideal weight and health goals.

Be Careful What You Ask For—You Just Might Get It

Whatever you ask for, by thinking about it repeatedly, especially with emotion, will be unconsciously accepted as important. Your brain will then begin to formulate action plans and stimulate automatic behaviors that will lead most expediently to you getting exactly what you were thinking about the most. However, this power is neutral and works in both directions.

The car was a positive goal, but what if something negative dominated your thinking? What if all day long you thought about what you didn't want? What if you focused on your fears? What if you worried about your health problems? What if you complained all day long about your physical limitations? What if you dwelt upon your need for a drink or comfort food? What if you complained about how much you hated being fat?

Most people focus on the negative, mull over their problems, and replay past failures in the theater of their minds. When you focus on what you don't want, you're programming your mind to get more of what you don't want.

If you download a virus onto your computer, it can erase your hard drive and your computer doesn't care—it's just running a program. Like a computer, your unconscious mind is totally impartial and will carry out whatever programming you install. Bad attitudes, limiting beliefs, and negative thinking are like thought viruses. If you install them in your brain by repeating statements such as "I'll always be fat" or "Nothing works for me," your unconscious doesn't evaluate whether your requests are good or bad. It simply follows instructions.

How Habits Are Developed and Strengthened

A habit is an automatic behavior pattern that has been turned over to unconscious control. Habits form because repeating a new behavior is like your conscious mind telling your unconscious mind, "Hey, I'm going to be doing this a lot, so let's make this easier to do next time and eventually make it automatic so I don't have to think about it anymore. I'm too busy with other things."

Dr. Richard Restak, a neurophsychiatrist and author of more than a dozen books about the human brain, explains that the more often you practice and re-peat something, the deeper the neural tracks and the easier it is to go down those tracks again in the future:

> **THIS PRINCIPLE OF REINFORCEMENT** through repetition has practical applica-tions for everyday life. For instance, if you want to learn a new skill or make use of new knowledge, you must change your brain. You must engage in repetitive exercises that set up the relevant circuits and sharpen their expression. This holds true what-ever your goal and whatever degree of mastery you seek.

You may have heard that it takes at least twenty-one to thirty days to develop a new habit. Functional MRI studies suggest that this timeworn self-help cliché is actually quite accurate. At the National Institutes of Health Laboratory for Brain and Cognition, researchers found that within three to four weeks of prac-ticing simple repetitive motor patterns, stronger neural pathways were devel-oped and there were also changes in three parts of the brain.

If the "twenty-one days to a new habit" advice is really true, then why do pos-itive new habits and healthy behaviors seem so hard to form? Shouldn't you be able to grunt it out for a few weeks with sheer willpower, and then eating healthy and working out will become as easy as driving your car? Well, that's ex-actly what would happen if it weren't for one problem: the old unconscious pro-gramming opposing your new conscious desires.

The solution is simple: reprogram your brain. When you embark on a program of mental training alongside your physical training, the old programming that could have sabotaged your new plan will weaken, new circuits will form, and your conscious desires and unconscious programming will come into alignment.

Goal Setting and Mental Reprogramming: A Scientific Approach

So far, we've established that your unconscious mind is a powerful goal-seeking computer, standing by at all times, waiting for your instructions. What's next?

First, you choose a target, then you program that target into your mind. It all starts with goal setting, the master skill of success. Because this process is based on neurology and psychology, not mysticism or metaphysics, I call it scientific goal setting. There are five simple steps.

STEP 1: Choose specific, measurable goals

The first step in achieving any goal is to answer the question "What do I want?" It seems straightforward enough, but the unconscious mind takes your requests literally and can't respond well to generalities, so you should be careful how you answer. If your goal is to lose weight, and if you sweat off one pound of water, then you've reached your goal. "Lose weight" is not a well-stated goal because it doesn't specify how much weight and which kind of weight you want to get rid of.

Clarity is power. Give your brain very specific targets, such as:

- How many pounds or kilos do you want to weigh?
- What body fat percentage do you want?
- What measurements would you like to have?
- What size clothes do you want to wear?

Describe your goals in as much detail as possible and be certain to use criteria that can be measured so there's no question about whether you've achieved them or not.

STEP 2: Set achievable goals but without limits

You may have set goals before, only to have your friends or family tell you to "be realistic." Setting healthy and achievable goals is important, but there are dangers in setting goals too low as well. Psychologist Abraham Maslow once said, "The story of the human race is the story of people selling themselves short."

Don't settle for anything less than what you really want. As long as your goal is achievable, believable, and you're willing to do what it takes to get it, then the sky's the limit.

Your goals are big enough if they're exciting and scary at the same time. If they're not, then you're staying inside your comfort zone and setting your goals too low. On the other hand, if you set a goal to drop fifteen pounds of pure body fat by next week, that's not optimism, it's self-delusion. Keep your fifteen-pound goal, but set a more appropriate deadline.

Almost all the top experts recommend reducing your weight by one or two pounds per week or no more than 1 percent of your total body weight per week. An achievable weekly body-fat percentage goal would be ½ percent per week. If you're an "overachiever," or you have more time for exercise than most people, then your results might be a little better. However, weight loss beyond two or three pounds per week is usually water or lean tissue.

When you set very specific goals, it's almost uncanny how often you hit them on the nose, right to the digit and to the day. This is proof of the power of clarity, but who's to say you may not have done better? The solution is to set goals with no limit. Setting "no limit" goals is as simple as adding a few extra words to your goal statement, such as "at least," "or more," "better," and so on.

For example, you might write, "I am burning at least ½ percent of body fat per week," or "My body fat percentage is dropping from 14 percent to 8 percent or lower." This gives you the best of both worlds because you've set a realistic goal, but it doesn't limit your level of achievement.

STEP 3: Set your goals with a deadline

In 1957, author Cyril Northcote Parkinson wrote for the first time about a powerful psychological principle: "Work expands to fill the time available for its completion." Parkinson's law, as it became widely known, explains the paradox of why the busiest people often get more accomplished than anyone else. It also reveals the power of deadlines. When you set realistic but challenging deadlines and keep them in the front of your mind, you're programming your brain to make the best use of every hour and to help you achieve more in less time.

Have you ever had an entire semester to write a research paper but you waited until the last minute, pulled an all-nighter, and barely got it turned in on the last day? Why is this experience so common? The closer the deadline, the higher the urgency. If you think you have plenty of time, there's less urgency.

Self-imposed deadlines are good, but externally imposed deadlines with built-in accountability and consequences for missing them are even better. In the case of a term paper, the consequence of not turning in the assignment on time is a failing grade and a permanent blemish on your report card. That might mean the pain of embarrassment, taking the course over again, or even a lower-paying job.

External deadlines with real rewards and real consequences increase your motivational leverage. To put it simply, they light a fire under your butt. For example, you could enroll in a before-and-after fitness transformation competition. When there's prize money and your photos will be seen by others, that provides tremendous drive to get in top shape.

I recommend setting your deadlines in five categories:

1. **Multiyear goals.** Start with a vision of your ultimate ideal physique. If you could have any body you wanted, what would that look like? Maybe it's an actor or movie star's physique. Maybe it's an athlete, bodybuilder, or fitness pro's body. Next, set long-term goals. Two to five years is the usual time frame. I've seen people go from obese to fitness model or bodybuilder in less than twenty-four months, so never sell yourself short when setting long-term goals. Finally, take an even longer perspective and set ten-, twenty-, and even fifty-year goals. How long do you plan to live? What will your body and health be like when you get older? What kind of activities will you be doing in your golden years?

2. **One-year goals.** Six months to a year is a midrange goal. When you have fifty to one hundred pounds or more to shed, midrange goals are especially important. Regardless of your objective or current fitness level, it's easy to think in terms of twelve-month periods and it's natural to set goals at the beginning of each calendar year, so be sure to take advantage of that.

3. **Twelve-week goals.** Early in the year, an annual goal deadline can seem so far away that it's easy to rationalize missing workouts or cheating on your diet and telling yourself it won't make a difference. With a twelve-week (short-term) goal deadline getting closer every day, you'll know that every workout and every meal counts. Your twelve-week goal is the one you should prioritize and focus on the most at any given time.

4. **Weekly goals.** Weekly goals let you break down your twelve-week goals into more manageable and easy-to-swallow chunks. Weekly body weight, body fat, and measurements are a phenomenal accountability tool. Weekly feedback is your progress report that tells you, "How am I doing?" It's the navigation system that tells you whether you're on target or in need of a course correction.

5. **Daily goals.** Daily goals may include outcomes for each workout such as weight lifted, reps performed, or calories burned. But they're also much more. Daily goals are the steps that you need to repeat every day to achieve your mid- and long-term goals. Doing three more reps of an exercise than you did at your last workout is a daily outcome goal. Eating a fruit or vegetable with every meal is a daily behavioral goal or action step.

For each time frame, write your goals in ink and your deadlines in pencil. The ink represents the fact that once you've set a goal for something you really want, never give up. Write your deadline in pencil as a reminder to keep your deadline flexible. If you don't make it in time, you didn't fail, you underestimated how long it would take. Simply erase that deadline, keep the goal, and set a new deadline.

STEP 4: Uncover your reasons

The simple act of setting a goal puts your brain's automatic pilot success mechanism to work for you. Goals, however, only give you a direction. Knowing the reasons you want your goals provides the motivation and drive that keep you moving in the right direction. Think of goals as the rudder and emotional reasons as the engine or propulsion system.

Each time you write down a goal, take a step beyond declaring what you want, and write down why you want it. Ask yourself, "What's important to me about this goal? What will achieving this goal do for me? What will be different when I have it? How will my life improve?" It's not the outcome of having a certain body fat percentage that really motivates you. It's what being leaner will do for you and how it will make you feel.

Most people say that being healthy is one of their reasons for wanting to lose weight. I believe that's a good choice, but unfortunately, their priorities are often out of order, with values such as "having a good time" placed above health. The proof is that many people won't make lifestyle changes unless they're threatened with a health problem. The health crisis then becomes the reason why and they're *forced* to move health to a higher rung in their hierarchy of values. If you choose health as one of your highest values, you'll probably never have to face a health crisis.

Next to health, family is usually at the top of the list. Beyond health and family, the reasons why each individual wants to get leaner and fitter are entirely personal and can range from sex appeal to spirituality. Here's a small sample of real reasons that I've heard from my clients over the years:

I want to:

- look good in my bikini for my trip to the Caribbean.
- be in perfect shape for my wedding and honeymoon.
- win the physique transformation contest I'm entering.
- look "hot" for my husband.
- feel more energetic.
- achieve perfect health.
- look in the mirror and like what I see.
- inspire other people with my own transformation.
- fit into the jeans I want to wear.
- look good naked.
- look ten years younger.
- live until I'm one hundred.
- honor my creator by treating my body like a temple.

● be a role model for my kids.

● be around to raise my kids and see my grandchildren.

● have more self-confidence and self-esteem.

● show everyone who said I was crazy and would never reach my goal that I did it.

When you set a goal and then connect that goal to your values, purpose, or reasons why, you'll never have trouble staying motivated again. The more reasons you have and the stronger the emotions around each reason, the more motivational horsepower you'll have propelling you toward your goal.

STEP 5: Write down your goals as affirmations

An idea, wish, or fantasy becomes a goal the instant you put it in writing. The act of writing helps put it on your brain's important list faster. Having your goals in writing also helps you use the power of repetition because you can read them repeatedly so they don't slip out of sight and out of mind.

The most effective way to write your goals is in a specific format called an affirmation, because this is the way your unconscious mind takes instructions the best. A powerful affirmation is written in the present tense, it's stated positively, and made personal.

● **Present tense.** Write all your goals as if you had already achieved them.

● **Personal.** Set goals for you, not for someone else, and be sure that you have control over the outcome.

● **Positive.** Set goals for what you want to get, not what you want to avoid or get rid of.

The first person pronoun *I* is a statement of personal identity, and some of your strongest beliefs are held at the identity level. "I am" affirmations can be very powerful. Other personal affirmations include: I have, I do, I eat, I exercise, I wear, I weigh, I enjoy, and so on.

Be sure to set goals as positives. Most people focus on weight loss. But if you say you want to lose weight, you didn't say what you wanted, you only said what you wanted to get rid of. The brain can't process negation. If I tell you, "Don't think about eating chocolate cake," you won't be able to do it. In fact, you're probably visualizing a piece of cake in your mind right now.

All around us in daily life there are endless examples of negative and counterproductive suggestions. A bad coach says, "Don't swing at the low outside pitches—you'll strike out." A good coach says, "When the right pitch comes, swing and knock that ball over the fence." The bad golfer says to himself, "Don't slice the ball into the sand trap." The good golfer says, "Hit it dead center of the green, right on top of the pin."

If you focus your attention on what you don't want, you're going to get more of it. Instead of losing weight, or getting rid of fat, state what you want, and be specific. Here are a few examples:

- I am feeling great on July 1, all my clothes fit loosely, my weight is under 185 pounds, and my body fat is now 10 percent or less.
- I am so happy and thankful now that I fit perfectly in my size 4 jeans by November 1 and looking so good in them when I wear them to work that I leave all the guys' jaws on the floor.
- By May 31, I weigh 125 pounds and my body fat percentage is less than 20 percent. I look awesome, feel great, and am ready for some summer fun.

Stating your goals as affirmations like these tells your brain in no uncertain terms exactly what you want. They are specific, measureable, personal, positive and deadline-driven.

Programming Your Goal into Your Mind with Spaced Repetition

If a goal remains a fleeting thought or conscious wish and you don't program it into your mind, then you won't follow through with the action steps necessary to achieve it. A perfect example is the New Year's resolution, a goal that's casually set and not reinforced, repeated, or emotionally driven into your brain. Therefore, it's taken as unimportant, quickly forgotten or abandoned as soon as the going gets tough. Repetition is one of the keys to retrain your brain.

Mental training should be scheduled, just like physical training. Commit to a specific time every morning right after you wake up and at night right before you fall asleep. This could be as little as five minutes if you're busy, or fifteen to twenty minutes or more if you're ambitious and have the time. Use these brief sessions to write new goals and review or rewrite your current goals. Rewriting your goals by hand every day is a powerful mental programming tool. I've had clients tell me that this one technique alone completely transformed their lives.

In addition to your morning and evening mind-training session, your objective is to flood your mind with positive images, words, sounds, thoughts, and feelings about what you want, from as many angles as possible, as often as possible throughout the day. Here are eight of the best ways to do it.

Eight Mental Training Tools to Program Your Unconscious Mind for Success

1. **Paper.** Goal setting can begin with nothing but a blank piece of paper and a pen. If you prefer, use 3 x 5 cards. Be sure to write down your outcome goals as well as a list of your daily behavioral goals. Although it's important to prioritize your goals and focus on the ones you consider most important, you can also write down all your goals in one master list. How many? As many as you can think of. Keep in mind that goal setting is not a one-time event, it's a process, a daily habit, and a discipline. Your goal lists will change and evolve as you change and evolve. As you review your lists every day, continue to rewrite and revise your affirmations until they sound just right. Continue adding new goals as you achieve the old ones.

2. **Goal card.** Choose the most important goal from your list (usually your twelve-week goal) and write it down as an affirmation on a wallet-size card.

Carry your goal card everywhere you go and read it constantly. Every time you open your wallet or your purse, or any time you have a few seconds to spare, such as in line at the bank or sitting in traffic, take out your card and read it. If you read your goal card often enough, you'll reach a point where even if you simply put your hands in your pocket and touch the card, it will make you think about your goal. This is a great way to stay focused and prioritize the one goal that's most important to you.

3. **Visualization and mental rehearsal.** When you visualize a skill, performance, or behavior in your mind, you're firing the same neurons in your brain as if you carried it out physically. This will prime your brain to help you carry out those behaviors in real life. Just as the athlete imagines him or herself flawlessly performing sports skills, you can imagine yourself taking the daily action steps necessary for reaching your perfect weight goal. Imagine yourself cooking and eating healthy, low-calorie foods, making better choices in restaurants, going to the gym consistently, or saying no to comfort foods in trigger situations. See yourself in your mind's eye already having the body you've always wanted. Visualizing your ideal body reprograms your self-image, which is the picture you have of yourself in your mind. When your self-image changes, your behavior changes to be consistent with that image.

4. **Photos.** Flip through some fitness magazines and cut out pictures of bodies that represent the ideal you'd like to have yourself. Even better, cut out a picture of your head and paste it on top of that photo of your ideal body. Try Photoshop to do it digitally and make it look realistic. This is also a great way to improve your visualization skills.

5. **Posters and signs.** Write down your goals on posters, signs, or notes and place them strategically throughout your kitchen, home, and office where you will see them often. Some people create a "vision board," which is a collage of various goal photos, affirmations, and motivational images pasted together on a bulletin board or poster board.

6. **Screen savers or pop-ups.** If you spend a lot of time in front of a computer, you can use pop-ups, sticky notes, or screen-saver software to have your

goals and affirmations appear on your screen at regular intervals. You can also use your desktop wallpaper to post your goals and goal-related images.

7. **Audios.** There are many excellent self-help, hypnosis, and motivational audios available for sale, which may be helpful with the mental reprogramming process. Perhaps even better is a personalized audio of your own goals and affirmations in your own voice. A great way to make your own audio is to string together a series of affirmations into a motivational script. Then read it into a computer microphone or digital voice recorder.

8. **Affirmations and self-talk.** Controlling your self-talk might be the single most powerful form of mental programming, due to the sheer number of thoughts you think every day. It's impossible to be positive 100 percent of the time, but "anti-negative" thinking may be even more important than positive thinking. Negative thoughts will pop up from time to time. So you should never beat yourself up for that. What matters is what you think about and focus on most of the time and how you talk back to that negative voice when it speaks up. You can challenge negative thoughts, you don't have to accept them.

To some people, these methods sound too simplistic to be so powerful. However, these techniques have been used for decades and proven effective by some of the most successful peak performers in history.

What's more, advances in neuroscience and clinical psychology have scientifically validated these techniques and shown us the reasons why they work. There are scientific laws of mind operating here. Think of gravity. Whether you believe in it or not doesn't stop it from working.

The High-Low Nutrition Solution

CHAPTER SIX

How to **Burn Fat** Automatically and **Feel Fuller** on **Less Food**

STUDIES suggest that the energy density of foods affects calorie intake, satiety, and ultimately body weight. Low-energy-density diets can help lower calorie intake without reducing food volume and thus help individuals avoid feeling hungry and deprived.

—BARBARA ROLLS, PH.D., PROFESSOR OF NUTRITIONAL SCIENCES, PENN STATE UNIVERSITY

You're about to learn how to get leaner, become healthier, and feel fuller even when you're eating less food. Using the simple nutrition rules in this chapter, you'll easily achieve your perfect weight and it won't seem like you're on a diet. Even better, you don't have to starve yourself or give up your favorite foods. You'll also have no problem maintaining your new body shape because you're not going to do anything weird or extreme to get there.

Getting leaner doesn't depend on fat grams, carbohydrate grams, meal timing, food combinations, macronutrient ratios, individual micronutrients, or any of a hundred other exotic diet program themes. None of those matter if you're eating too much. In the end, nearly every weight-loss strategy comes back full circle to whether it helps you maintain a calorie deficit.

Staying in a calorie deficit consistently, however, is a challenge because so many variables influence how much you eat and how many calories you burn. Energy balance is dynamic, which means the amount of calories you require can change. Next to underestimating food consumption, forgetting to adjust your calorie intake when your energy needs change is the most common cause of weight-loss plateaus.

The big question is, "What is the most painless, efficient, and healthiest way to maintain that vital caloric deficit?" For my money, I'll bet on what I call "high-low" nutrition, an approach to food selection based on three important principles:

1. **Energy density**, also known as calorie density, is the number of calories in a food per serving.
2. **Nutrient density** is the nutritional value per serving (vitamins, minerals, phytonutrients, and fiber).
3. **Satiety** is how full a food or meal makes you feel and how that affects how much you eat.

To maximize fat loss while optimizing your health, your goal is to choose foods that contain the highest nutrient density, the highest satiety value, and the lowest calorie density.

Is a Calorie Just a Calorie?

You may be thinking, "There's a lot more to nutrition than just calories, and a calorie is not just a calorie!" Precisely. That's the whole point of eating nutrient-dense, natural foods. Obviously, 200 calories from pretzels and soda won't provide the same nutritional value or satiating power as 200 calories of broccoli and salmon. Different foods can profoundly affect your health, your hormones, and even your mood, alertness, and mental function.

Different types of foods can also have slightly different effects on body composition at the same gross caloric intake. This can be explained by the thermic effect of food, calories in fibrous foods that aren't completely absorbed, and the effect of food on hormones and subsequent appetite. But this doesn't disprove the calorie law, it verifies it. Accounting for all these factors, when you look at the net result, you're left with exactly what the math dictates: body mass changes are based on calories in versus calories out. From an energy balance point of view, a metabolizable calorie is just a calorie.

There's a big difference between "don't count calories" and "calories don't count." Some diet programs discourage calorie counting; they simply tell you what to eat and what not to eat. The special food combinations or unique theme of the diet are usually credited for the weight loss. What they don't tell you is that their eating rules make you eat less automatically.

A Different Definition of Counting Calories

At this point you may be thinking, "Oh no, not another calorie-counting program!" If so, take a deep breath. You won't have to count calories forever. In fact, if you're adamant about not counting anything, I won't insist on it. I'll simply ask you to do three things:

1. Acknowledge the calories-in versus calories-out equation.
2. Be aware of your portion sizes.
3. Increase or decrease your portions in response to your weekly results.

My definition of counting calories may not be what you think. Counting calories doesn't have to mean walking around with a notebook or electronic device, writing down every morsel you eat throughout each day. Instead, you create a daily menu plan as your eating goal for the day.

Using this method, you only need to count calories once when you create your menu. This method is proactive, not reactive. You write down what you plan to eat first, then eat it, rather than eating first and then writing down what you just ate. Think of it as menu planning rather than calorie counting. To prevent boredom and get nutritional variety, you can create multiple menus or make food substitutions from the same category with similar caloric values.

Making your own menus is easier than you think. Simply follow the ten Body Fat Solution nutrition rules and your menus will almost create themselves. For a fast start, use the food lists in the Appendix.

CALORIES 101: Calculate Your Daily Maintenance Calories

One size does not fit all when it comes to calories. It's silly to prescribe the same amount of calories for everyone, especially if it lumps men and women or active and sedentary people together. For example, 1,500 calories a day might be optimal for most women to reduce fat, but it could be semistarvation for a large, highly active man.

The bigger and more active you are, the more calories you need to maintain your weight. Remember these points and that both can change. Also keep in mind that women are generally smaller than men, so women usually need about 600 to 800 fewer calories each day. Calorie needs also decrease as you get older.

According to exercise physiologists Victor Katch and Frank McArdle, the average female between the ages of twenty-three and fifty has a maintenance level of about 2,000 to 2,100 calories per day and the average male about 2,700 to 2,900 calories.

CALORIES 102: Create the All-important Calorie Deficit

To shed fat, you must create a caloric deficit. A caloric deficit, also known as negative energy balance, means that the number of calories you consume is less than the number of calories you burn. You can create a deficit by decreasing your food intake, increasing your activity level, or both. If you require 2,800 calories per day to maintain your weight and you eat 3,300 calories per day, you're in positive energy balance by 500 calories and you'll gain weight. If you eat 2,300 calories per day, you're in negative energy balance and you'll lose weight.

A caloric deficit is simple subtraction. To calculate your ideal caloric intake for reducing body fat, subtract 20–30 percent from your maintenance level. Twenty percent is considered a conservative deficit; 30 percent, an aggressive deficit.

If you're an average male and your maintenance level is 2,800 calories per day, then a 20 percent deficit is a 560-calorie reduction, which gives you a goal of 2,240 calories per day. If you're an average female and your maintenance level is 2,100 calories per day, then a 20 percent deficit is 1,680 calories per day.

It's generally best to keep your calorie reduction conservative at first. If you're not getting the rate of fat loss you want, you can create a more aggressive deficit later by reducing your calories a little further or increasing your activity.

On average, most women will reduce body fat effectively and safely on 1,400 to 1,800 calories per day. Most men will achieve healthy, safe, and effective fat reduction on about 2,100 to 2,500 calories per day. Remember that these are averages. If your body is large and you're active, use the upper end of these ranges. If your body is small or you're inactive, use the lower end of these ranges.

CALORIES 103: Adjust Your Calorie Intake or Exercise Output on the Basis of Your Results

There are many formulas you can use to calculate your calorie needs with precision. However, don't be overly concerned about calorie calculations, because you'll have to adjust your calories based on your weekly results anyway. All you need is a good baseline. In the end, it's more important that you understand the big picture of energy balance.

Regardless of the number of calories you think you're eating right now, if your body weight is not changing, then you don't have a calorie deficit. This means one of three things:

1. You underestimated how many calories you are eating.
2. You overestimated how many calories you are burning.
3. Both of the above.

Whatever the reason, you need to create or reestablish a deficit by eating less or exercising more.

The Selective Reduction of Calories

There are two ways to create a deficit: increase your energy expenditure or decrease your food consumption. On the food reduction side, the next question is, "Which foods do you cut?" Do you simply eat a little less of everything? That would work, because any caloric deficit will cause weight loss. But there's a better way.

First, establish a balanced and sensible baseline by following the ten Body Fat Solution nutrition rules. Then, when a decrease in calories is called for, you selectively reduce the calorie-dense simple sugars, starchy carbs, and grains. That leaves the essential proteins, fats, and micronutrients from fruits and vegetables relatively untouched. If the calories fall too low to satisfy your energy needs, you simply add caloric ballast by slightly increasing your lean protein and healthy fats.

If you're an astute reader, you might be thinking, "Hey, wait a minute, aren't you creating another low-carb diet in disguise?" Well, yes and no. Yes, because we're increasing your caloric deficit by reducing certain carbs. No, because there are some important differences in my approach compared to "traditional" low-carb diets:

● First, this eating plan is not an extreme low-carb diet, it's a moderate-carb nutrition program.
● Second, the amount of carbs you reduce is not fixed, it's a variable based on your needs and preferences.
● Third, the type of carbs you eliminate right from the start are the processed

carbs, refined sugars, and man-made carbs. As results dictate, you also reduce natural starches and grains, which are calorie dense. There's no reason to remove high-nutrient-density foods like fruits and veggies.

- Fourth, the primary focus is not on carbs, but where it should be—on the calories.

Traditional low-carb dieting mentality can sometimes lead to the misunderstanding and condemnation of perfectly healthy and nutritious foods and makes carbs look like the cause of obesity. The cause of obesity is not carbs, it's an excess of calories, a decrease in physical activity, and all the factors that lead to this energy imbalance.

The Macronutrients: Protein, Carbohydrates, and Fat

Like calories, the proper intake of the three macronutrients—proteins, healthy carbs, and essential fats—is critical. However, if you simply follow the ten Body Fat Solution nutrition rules, your macronutrient needs will be met and you'll automatically be in the ballpark with all your numbers. What's most important is to get the essentials first and find a healthful macronutrient balance that avoids the extremes. From there, you can customize the plan to meet your needs.

Before we move on to the ten rules, let's briefly overview the three macronutrients.

The Power of Protein

The word "protein" comes from the Greek *proteos*, which means "of first importance." This is appropriate because when you prepare a meal, I want you to think of lean protein first. Think of protein as building material for the body because the amino acids in protein are used as construction material for nearly every cell and tissue, including muscle.

Protein is found in many foods, even vegetables, beans, legumes, and whole grains. While this is important for vegetarians to know, when we refer to "lean proteins" in this program, we're referring primarily to the lean sources of complete proteins, ones that contain all the essential amino acids. Complete proteins include chicken breast, turkey breast, lean red meat, fish, shellfish, egg whites, and low- or nonfat dairy products.

Protein plays some very important roles in weight control. Lean protein helps you maintain your lean body mass when your calories are restricted. It also helps suppress your appetite.

Eating lean protein increases your metabolism due to the thermic effect of food, which is how much energy you burn to digest the food. Protein has a thermic effect of 30 percent. This means that if you eat a lean protein food that has 100 calories, 30 of those calories are used to digest and process the food, leaving only 70 calories of net energy available. Carbohydrates have a thermic effect of 10–15 percent, while dietary fat has the lowest thermic effect of only 3 percent.

An important research review published in the *Journal of the American College of Nutrition* succinctly summed up the power of protein. The study, titled "The Effects of High Protein Diets on Thermogenesis, Satiety and Weight Loss," said:

THERE IS CONVINCING EVIDENCE that a higher protein intake exerts an increased thermic effect when compared to fat and carbohydrate. Evidence is also convincing that higher protein diets increase satiety when compared to lower protein diets. In dietary practice, it may be beneficial to partially replace refined carbohydrates with protein sources that are low in saturated fat.

Calories count, but a calorie is not just a calorie, especially when it comes to protein calories.

Carbohydrates

When you think of carbs, think of fuel or energy. You're always burning a mix of fat and carbohydrate, as if you were a car with two fuel tanks. At times, however, you burn more of one fuel or the other. Carbs are your body's primary fuel source during intense physical activity. Fat is your primary fuel at rest and during low-intensity activity. If you're doing a lot of vigorous training, you're going to need more carbs for maximum performance. If you're lightly active or sedentary, you can get by with eating fewer carbs.

For body fat management and optimal health, it's important to divide carbs into several categories because not all carbs are created equal.

Processed carbs—limit or avoid. Man-made or refined carbohydrates include white sugar (sucrose), white flour, high-fructose corn syrup, and any other highly processed sugars. They usually come in boxes, packages, cans, or wrappers. The processed carbs, especially "the whites"—sugar and flour—have a low nutrient density, which is why they're called "empty calories." They also have a high calorie density, which is why they contribute to excess body fat.

Whole grains and natural starches—eat in small to moderate quantities. Natural 100 percent whole grains (whole wheat, barley, rye, oats, spelt, quinoa) and natural starches (potatoes, yams, brown rice, beans, legumes) can play an important role in a body-fat-reducing program. Natural grains and starches are high in nutrient density and help to fuel your workouts. Many are also high in fiber, which is beneficial for health, appetite control, and body-fat reduction. The only downside is that they're also higher in energy density than fibrous carbs. If you want to reduce your body fat, adjust your intake of starchy carbs and grains according to your calorie budget, activity level, and state of metabolic health.

Fibrous carbs and nonstarchy vegetables—eat in large quantities. Green vegetables and nonstarchy vegetables, also known as fibrous carbs, are nutritional champions because they're the type of carbs with the lowest energy density and the highest nutrient density. Vegetables are a win-win proposition because they benefit you in terms of health as well as fat reduction.

Fruit and natural simple carbs—eat in moderate quantities. Fruit is another natural source of carbs, with low to moderate energy density and very high nutrient density. It's odd that some people believe fruit is fattening, but it's probably because of confusion about fruit sugar. Fruit contains a natural sugar called fructose, which is processed differently in the body than other carbs. Fructose in whole fruit is not the same thing as the high-fructose corn syrup found in many soft drinks and processed foods. In any case, it's not fructose that makes you fat, it's an excess of calories.

Carbs are not inherently fattening outside of their ability to easily deliver an excess of calories, if you choose the wrong ones. A little-known fact in this age of "carbo-phobia" is that carbs are rarely converted to body fat.

Our rationale for moderating carbs is different than conventional low-carb dogma: Reducing sugars, starches, and grains, while keeping fibrous carbs, healthy fats, and lean proteins more or less constant, does help control insulin. But more important, it's simply one of the better ways to keep your calories under control while retaining all the nutritional essentials.

Fat

There is a good reason why I gave you a lecture about dietary fat myths in Chapter Two. If you harbor a strong belief that eating dietary fat makes you fat, you're likely to miss out on one of the most healthful and important nutrients—the essential fatty acids (EFAs). EFAs are so named because they're necessary for human health and normal growth. They must be obtained from the foods you eat because your body can't make them.

The richest animal source of EFAs is fatty fish. Fatty fish contains two important long-chain polyunsaturated omega-3 fatty acids called eicosapentaenoic acid (EPA) and docosahexaenoic acid (DHA). These are the major players responsible for the biological activity in fish oil. Recent studies suggest that omega-3 essential fatty acids from fish can help optimize the fat-burning process. Omega-3 fats are also extremely heart healthy.

The richest plant source of omega-3 is flaxseed oil. You can also get omega-3 from walnuts, some seeds, and small amounts from dark leafy greens. The oil from flaxseed also contains large amounts of LNA, alpha-linolenic acid, the plant-based omega-3 fatty acid. The other healthy fat is the monounsaturated variety, which includes sources such as extra-virgin olive oil, olives, avocados, and almonds.

Human beings evolved on a diet that was free of man-made trans-fatty acids and lower in saturated fatty acids than the modern diet. It also contained roughly equal amounts of omega-3 and omega-6 fatty acids. The modern Western diet today is very high in omega-6 relative to omega-3, with a ratio of 20:1 or even higher. Most people don't consume enough healthy fats, and their omega-3 to omega-6 ratio is skewed badly in favor of the pro-inflammatory omega-6.

One of the reasons for this imbalance is a decrease in fish consumption and an increase in the use of refined oils. The industrial production of animal feeds, which contain grains high in omega-6 fatty acids, have also produced beef and poultry with an undesirable fatty acid composition. In addition to eating more fatty fish, choosing grass-fed beef, omega-3 eggs, and fewer refined grains can also help correct this problem.

For decades, saturated fats, the kind found in meat and butter, were red-flagged as the bad fats to avoid. However, there's an ongoing controversy over the saturated fat, cholesterol, and heart disease connection. It's been proposed that saturated fats may not be the bad guys they were made out to be. Although the subject is still being debated, it's clear that the effect of saturated fat may vary based on the type of saturated fat, as well as your current health status, genetic predispositions, and what else you eat every day.

Nevertheless, in most cases, saturated fats should probably make up only a small part of your daily fat intake, if for no other reason than to leave room in your calorie budget for the healthy fats, lean proteins, and natural carbs. The key is a balance between the saturated, polyunsaturated, and monounsaturated fats, with an emphasis on natural food sources, not the demonization and elimination of all saturates.

Trans-fatty acids, on the other hand, are unnatural fats used to prolong the shelf life and increase commercial uses of processed foods. Avoid these as much as possible. Trans fats have been linked to cardiovascular disease and some experts believe there is no safe level of intake. In a recent study from Wake Forest University, researchers found that trans-fatty acids may also cause an increase in intraabdominal body fat, and increased insulin resistance.

Trans fats are found in baked goods, fried foods, and packaged convenience foods such as cookies, crackers, biscuits, pies, frostings, pastries, doughnuts, corn chips, taco shells, margarine, shortening, and French fries. The dead giveaway of a trans fat is to read the ingredients label on food products and look for "hydrogenated" and "partially hydrogenated" oils.

The Ten Body Fat Solution Nutrition Rules

After more than twenty years of designing nutrition programs that counted every food to the calorie and gram, I've reached some important conclusions.

First, counting calories and grams, calculating nutrient ratios, and weighing or measuring food is extremely effective because it removes most of the guesswork. Second, it lets you easily pinpoint problems. You can't troubleshoot something very well unless you've quantified and tracked it first. Third, putting it on paper helps to improve compliance by increasing personal accountability. Fourth, it provides an education in nutrition and food values that can't be equaled any other way.

For all the virtues of precisely calculating calories, macronutrient ratios, and grams of protein, carbs, and fat, there are downsides. Number crunching can be tedious, time-consuming work, even with the Internet, software, or handheld electronic devices. It's not an exact science and most people don't have the patience or inclination to do it. I'll always be in favor of doing "nutrition by the numbers." However, my goal for the Body Fat Solution program was to make nutrition a breeze for the average busy person who demands simplicity, practicality, and results at the same time.

By giving you simple nutrition rules that you can understand and apply on the level of daily behaviors, I can show you how to get your nutritional numbers not only in the ballpark, but remarkably close to your optimal target, without turning it into a science project or math equation.

These guidelines appear simple, but they're the result of boiling down over two decades of scientific research and hands-on experience. What follows are ten action steps that bring healthy, fat-burning nutrition to the level of everyday lifestyle.

1. Focus on the calorie deficit first and budget calories wisely

You could follow every rule of good nutrition, but if you're eating more calories than your body can use, then the excess will be stored as fat. Yes, even healthy, nutrient-dense food will cause weight gain if you eat too much of it. Every time you eat, the first question you have to ask is how many calories your meal contains. When faced with a choice between two foods or meals, choose the one lower in calories.

Saying calories arc the main thing doesn't imply they're the only thing. People who get a large percentage of their calories from processed foods might stay slim by keeping their portions small, but that doesn't mean they'll be healthy.

Always keep processed foods to a minimum to allow room for healthier, more nutrient-rich foods. For every junk-food calorie you include in your limited-calorie budget, another clean-food calorie gets pushed out or displaced. If it's not displaced, then adding junk food increases your calorie surplus or shrinks your deficit.

The lower your caloric intake, the more important it is to budget calories carefully. Your first priorities are essential amino acids (protein), essential fats, and foods rich in essential vitamins and minerals (vegetables and fruits). Eating low-nutrient junk foods while you're in a caloric deficit is like buying a trip around the world when you're having trouble paying the rent. It's a luxury you can't afford.

Every day you must look at your calorie intake the same way you'd look at your financial budget. Ask yourself, "What's the best way to spend my calories?" For example, if you're on a 1,500-calorie daily meal plan, do you really want to spend 500 of those calories—one-third of your intake—on a few sodas or alcoholic drinks, and leave only 1,000 for health-promoting food, fiber, and lean muscle-building protein? I realize some people may say yes to that, but then again, if some people spent their money as frivolously as they spent their calories, they'd be in the poorhouse in no time.

Anytime you're unsure whether you should eat a particular food, pause before eating and ask yourself these questions:

1. How many calories are in this food? Is it high or low in calorie density?
2. Does this food have nutritional "plus" value that will improve my health?
3. Does this food have nutritional "minus" value that will damage my health?
4. Is this a good way to spend my calories right now?
5. Can I afford it?

2. Start building every meal with lean protein

Start each meal by picking any food from the lean protein group. This includes eggs (eat the yolks in moderation due to the high calorie density), turkey breast, chicken breast, lean red meat, bison, game meats, fish, shellfish, and also high-protein dairy products such as low- or nonfat cottage cheese, cheese, milk, or yogurt. Protein supplements such as whey, casein, or mixes of both can also make protein nutrition easier.

Protein is vital when your calories are restricted. Protein protects you from losing muscle, it decreases your appetite and makes you feel fuller. Many of the body composition benefits attributed to low-carb diets are actually benefits of higher protein intake.

My goal is to give you guidelines that help keep you away from number crunching as much as possible. However, the two numbers that are most important are calories and protein. Traditional recommendations for protein were developed for sedentary populations to avoid deficiency. The guidelines you'll use are designed for healthy people who are doing cardio and weight training while optimizing fat-burning results on a calorie-restricted program.

Research on the ideal numbers in this scenario suggests 0.8 to 1.0 grams of protein per pound of target body weight every day. Even more may be called for in certain cases such as bodybuilding and intense strength training. Prescribing protein by grams per pound of total body weight may overestimate protein needs in people with high body fat levels. That's why our recommendation is based on grams per pound of target body weight. Although macronutrient percentages must be viewed as relative based on total caloric intake, this usually comes out to 30–40 percent of total calorie intake. The other 60–70 percent of the calories will come from natural carbs and healthy fats.

What are the implications of this protein rule if you're vegetarian? Not to worry. Humans are omnivores, which means you can get lean and healthy with meat or without it. A two-year randomized trial was recently completed at the University of North Carolina comparing a total vegetarian diet with a more moderate diet. After the one- and two-year checkpoints, the vegan dieters had lost more weight than the group that had eaten a low-fat nonvegetarian diet.

The researchers in this study emphasized: "The primary mechanism by which a vegan diet leads to a reduction in body weight is a reduction in dietary energy density, due to its low fat and high fiber content." Meaning the vegetarians ate less automatically. Once again, we come back to calories and we see that even the vegetarian versus meat-eater debate takes a backseat to energy-in versus energy-out considerations.

If you're a vegetarian, then you can simply substitute the animal protein for a vegetarian protein such as soy, tofu, tempeh, or complementary proteins from mixing and matching vegetable proteins.

3. Eat vegetables (fibrous carbs) with every meal

Eat at least five to six servings of fibrous (nonstarchy) carbs a day, one for every meal or snack, or two different veggies for each main meal. In an ideal day, every meal would include one or more of the following:

- **Green vegetables** such as broccoli, asparagus, artichokes, green beans, collard greens, spinach, celery, Brussels spouts, or peas, which are starchy, but low in energy density.
- **Salad vegetables** such as leafy greens, tomatoes, cucumbers, radishes, or peppers.
- **Any other fibrous vegetables,** including mushrooms, onions, zucchini, squash, eggplant, beets, cauliflower, water chestnuts, cabbage, or carrots, which are starchy, but low in energy density.

As the name implies, most fibrous vegetables are high in fiber. Fiber plays an important role in maintaining a healthy digestive system, as it keeps things moving through the plumbing smoothly. Fiber is also known to reduce the risk of chronic diseases, including heart disease and some types of cancer, and it may help lower total and HDL cholesterol. Fiber also decreases the digestion rate of carbohydrates and helps manage blood sugar levels.

Greens and fibrous vegetables are densely loaded with vitamins, minerals, and health-promoting phytochemicals that provide many amazing benefits. Fibrous and green veggies have a very high nutrient density but very low calorie density and are highly satiating, the ultimate combination. Most veggies and greens are so low in calorie density, they could almost be considered "unlimited" foods because it's virtually impossible to overeat them.

A great breakfast tip is to make egg scrambles or omelets that are loaded with all kinds of fibrous and nonstarchy vegetables such as mushrooms, onions, green or red peppers, and tomatoes, along with your favorite spices. They are incredibly filling and satisfying.

A great lunch or dinner tip is to eat your lean protein and fill up on salad and veggies before eating any of the calorie-dense grains or starchy carbs. Research has shown that you're more likely to spontaneously eat less if you fill up on low-energy-density carbs first. Trading the bread basket and fried appetizers for a first-course salad (without the high-calorie toppings) is an easy way to reduce your calories and increase your fat loss with one simple substitution.

4. Eat omega-3 and other healthy fats every day

There's no need to obsessively cut fat out of your diet. Dietary fat does not cause more body fat storage at the same caloric intake. However, since fat has the highest calorie density at 9 calories per gram, it does have the potential to lead to excessive calorie consumption. Although eating dietary fat is satisfying psychologically due to its richness, the latest research shows that physiologically, it's really protein and high-fiber foods that are most satiating.

The best approach for long-term success is to avoid extremes of high- or low-fat diets. Instead, aim for a healthy balance between protein, carbs, and fat and between monounsaturated, polyunsaturated, and saturated fats. Your goal is to eat omega-3 fats every day and include a total of up to two or three servings of healthy fat per day.

Omega-3 fatty acids are among the "big three essentials," which include essential fats, essential micronutrients (vitamins and minerals), and essential amino acids (from lean proteins). One of the best ways to get your omega-3s is from fatty fish and other marine sources. Salmon and sardines, for example, are loaded with healthy omega-3 fats. You can also obtain omega-3 fats from vegetable sources such as ground flaxseed, walnuts, and dark leafy greens.

If you eat a meal that's inherently low fat, such as a lettuce and raw vegetable salad with chicken breast, then you could add some healthy fats to that meal. An olive oil dressing (healthy monounsaturated fat), avocado, or some chopped walnuts (healthy omega-3 polyunsaturated fats) would all work. Sometimes, the healthy fat is already in your food. For example, if you eat salmon with dinner, you not only get lean protein, you also get essential fats along with it. If you don't eat fish, or if most of the foods you eat are very low in fat, then it makes sense to add extra fats in the form of an essential fatty acid supplement such as fish oil or flaxseed oil.

5. Eat at least two fruits every day

Like vegetables, fruits are nutritional powerhouses, loaded with vitamins and health-promoting phytochemicals. Fruit is also a great source of fiber. Blueberries, blackberries, strawberries, raspberries, pears, peaches, cantaloupes, grapes, pineapples, papayas, bananas, grapefruits, nectarines, oranges, and apples are just some of the fantastic fruits you can choose from that are high in fiber, high in nutrients, and low in calories.

Although most fruits have a slightly higher caloric density than fibrous vegetables, with an average piece containing only 60 to 90 calories, they're mostly low-calorie foods compared to calorie-dense starches, grains, and processed sugars. Be aware that some fruits are more calorie dense than others. Bananas average about 120 calories each. Because of the low water content, dried fruits are extremely calorie dense. Raisins, for example, have 260 calories in a mere half cup. When you're on a tight calorie budget, use dried fruits only in very small quantities or avoid them in favor of fresh fruit.

I recommend you eat at least two fruits a day, and more if you're highly active and can fit them into your calorie budget. Include them with meals, on the side with lunch or breakfast, or as snacks between meals. Be sure to eat a wide variety of different fruits of every color over the course of each week.

6. Eat natural starches and grains as your "X-factor"

Once you have the essentials in place—lean proteins, healthy fats, and fibrous vegetables and fruits—you'll probably have room left in your calorie budget for another group of carbs, the natural starches and natural grains. The word "natural" is an important distinction because white carbs (white-sugar and white-flour products) and processed grains are not the same and should not be on your regular food lists.

Many low-carb diets require the elimination of all starchy carbs and grains, even if they're natural in origin, high in fiber, high in nutrients, and low in calories. This is not necessary. Instead of demonizing starches and grains, you should make natural starches and grains your nutritional X-factor. This means that while lean protein, healthy fat, and fibrous carbs remain relatively constant in your daily nutrition, the natural starches and grains should be a variable.

How much of this X-factor you consume depends on several other variables. First is exercise. The harder and more often you train, the more of these concentrated carbs you can afford to consume. One of the best times to consume your starches, higher-calorie carbs, and simple sugars is immediately after your workout, when your body needs the nutrients quickly for replenishment. Here's a simple way to remember this rule: "You haven't earned it until you've burned it."

Even if you have a preference for lower-carb nutrition, I recommend including at least one serving of natural starches or whole grains in your daily menu. Eat them with your breakfast to help reduce hunger and cravings later in the day (natural oatmeal is a great choice). On workout days, the ideal time for calorie-dense carbs is after your workouts, even if you train at night.

Remember that carbs have an important place in post-workout and sports nutrition. The more active you are, the more carbs you can utilize. Furthermore, some people, especially obese and sedentary individuals, appear "carbohydrate intolerant" from a health perspective. But many others metabolize carbohydrates perfectly, especially when they're maintaining a caloric deficit, exercising, and dropping weight.

Your X-factor could include multiple daily servings of natural starches and grains—it's all based on your energy needs, your state of metabolic health, and your weekly results. When you need to create a greater deficit, do it by selectively reducing your X-factor. When you need to increase your energy needs, do it by selectively increasing your X-factor.

If you can't eat whole-wheat products due to allergies or intolerances, that's not a problem; you can stick with the fibrous carbs and fruits. You could also explore some lesser-known types of natural whole grains, such as spelt or quinoa.

7. Eat mostly foods that pass the "natural test"

From a health and body fat perspective, the single most important criterion for choosing which carbohydrates and other foods to eat is whether they're natural or processed. Perhaps carbs and fats aren't the issue after all. Maybe the real problem is unnatural man-made carbs and fats. When deciding what foods to eat, the ultimate solution is to ask the "natural food question."

DID THIS FOOD come directly from a tree, from a plant, from out of the ground, or did it walk, fly, or swim?

If the answer is yes, then it's natural. (If you're vegetarian, you're welcome to use only the first half of our natural definition.)

Most of the time, processed foods are easy to identify, as they're usually found in boxes, cans, cartons, packages, or wrappers. Sometimes what's natural is not as obvious, so you need to read food labels and think it through carefully.

You've seen an orange tree, but you've never seen an orange-juice tree. Durum semolina from pasta is processed from wheat, which grows from the ground, but there's no such thing as a pasta plant. Even a lot of health foods don't meet our criteria for natural. There are "nutrition" bars you can get at the natural foods store, but have you ever seen a protein bar hanging from a branch? They're all manufactured.

After asking the "natural question," you'll be left primarily with lean meats, fish, shellfish, fruits, fibrous vegetables, salad vegetables, root vegetables, legumes, beans, nuts, seeds, and natural starches such as brown rice, yams, potatoes, and sweet potatoes. For the most part, this is what human beings ate before the arrival of modern food processing.

Some foods, such as 100 percent whole grains, aren't highly refined, but they're processed into breads, cereals, and pastas with the whole grain still intact. You could easily include some whole-grain bread, cereal, or pasta in moderation. However, consider these lightly processed carbs as second choices. Prioritize the foods that are as close to their natural form as possible.

8. Eat five to six times a day—a meal or a snack every three hours

Eating five to six small meals daily is the preferred method of many athletes and bodybuilders. It's arguably the optimal way to fuel a highly active person, especially someone who wants to build muscle or maintain high levels of physical performance. It's also a good way to help control appetite and manage blood sugar levels. However, some people find cooking, meal preparation, and eating every three hours too difficult of a lifestyle commitment.

Because snacks don't require time-consuming meal preparation or cooking, the easiest meal plan is three traditional meals a day—breakfast, lunch, and dinner—with snacks in between. This suits a busy lifestyle and helps improve compliance. If you prefer, you can eat like an athlete and divide your calories evenly into five or six small meals. This approach makes good sense when your calorie needs are high. What's most important is following a consistent eating schedule every day rather than eating haphazardly, because this allows you to develop a baseline.

A Body Fat Solution program meal contains a lean protein, as well as one or two natural carbs. A snack can be as simple as a piece of fruit, yogurt, a handful of nuts, or a protein shake. When choosing snacks, if you remember to ask the natural food question, you instantly remove a lot of undesirable snacks in one fell swoop. Instead of packaged, processed snack foods, try these nine power snacks instead:

- nuts and seeds (almonds, walnuts, sunflower seeds, and so on);
- raw vegetables;
- fruit;
- yogurt;
- cheese;
- cottage cheese;
- lean proteins (sardines, hard-boiled eggs, sliced turkey breast, canned fish, canned chicken);
- protein shakes and high-protein meal replacement shakes;
- soup made from natural ingredients.

An ideal snack would include protein, but since eating meat or fish for snacks may not be practical, aim for at least one protein snack per day. Dairy products such as cottage cheese, cheese, and yogurt all contain complete protein, so unless you are lactose-intolerant, these make good snack choices. If you choose the low- or nonfat varieties, that will help keep the calorie density low.

If you snack on nuts, be careful of serving sizes, because nuts are a high-nutrient-density, high-energy-density food. They give you lots of valuable nutrients, but also lots of calories because they are high in fat and low in water content.

Soup makes a good snack and can even be used as a primary meal or part of a meal. Research shows that soup is more satiating than other types of liquid calories.

9. Limit or avoid liquid calories and drink mostly water or green tea instead

Liquid beverages such as soda are high-calorie-density, zero-nutrient-density foods—the worst possible kind. They also don't activate the satiety mechanisms in your brain, stomach, and GI tract the way they do when you eat, chew, and swallow whole foods.

If you accounted for your calories meticulously, you could drink calorie-containing beverages and still reduce your body fat. However, the caloric density of many beverages is high and it's too easy to unconsciously consume an enormous amount of calories quickly by drinking them. Dessert coffees are quickly catching up to soda as one of the most common fattening beverages by virtue of extremely high calorie density.

Alcohol is problematic because it has the second-highest calorie density at 7 calories per gram. Some evidence says that one drink of red wine per day may offer health benefits. Alcohol, however, does not help your fat-reducing efforts because alcohol adds empty calories or displaces nutritious calories. While alcohol is being metabolized, fat oxidation is almost completely halted.

To maximize fat-burning results, drink few, if any, of your calories. If you use any liquid meal replacements, be sure to account for all the liquid calories and consider making thick shakes, which contain ingredients that have some degree of "chew factor." Avoid soda. Drink alcohol in moderation or not at all. Eat whole fruit instead of drinking fruit juice.

Coffee is acceptable in moderation, as long as you don't add a lot of calories to it from milk, cream, whipped cream, sugar, flavorings, and syrups. Green tea is an outstanding beverage because it's loaded with antioxidants and other health-promoting compounds.

Most of all, drink water. An individualized guideline that accounts for your activity level is the National Research Council's recommendation of 1.0 to 1.5 ml per calorie expended. For the average female, that's 1.9 to 2.9 liters (66 to 100 ounces) a day and for the average male, about 2.7 to 4.1 liters (93 to 139 ounces) daily. If you're an athlete or you exercise in the heat, aim for the higher end of these ranges. Keep in mind that this guideline includes total water from all sources and that it's entirely possible to drink too much water. More is not better.

10. Follow the 90/10 compliance rule

Depriving yourself completely of your favorite foods is unnecessary. It's also counterproductive because you crave what you're not allowed to have. After a while, the cravings build up to the point of losing control. If you're obsessed with thoughts about food, you're out of balance. On the Body Fat Solution program, there are no forbidden foods. Instead, you'll use a compliance rule.

Compliance refers to how many of your meals adhere to the rules of the program. The premise is that if you follow the rules 90 percent of the time, then what you eat the other 10 percent of the time won't matter much. But it will release you from the guilt of occasional indulgences and take the pressure of perfection off your shoulders.

Based on my experience with thousands of personal coaching clients, I've found a 90 percent compliance approach far more effective than allowing an entire cheat day. A full cheat day wouldn't be a bad idea, except that many people interpret that as permission for an anything-goes binge day.

I also suggest calling your 10 percent meals "free meals" instead of cheat meals because cheating presupposes it's something you're not supposed to do. If the 10 percent rule is part of the program to begin with, then it's not cheating, right? When you cheat, you feel guilty. Guilt is one of the strongest negative emotions and biggest diet destroyers.

Body Fat Solution Nutrition in a Nutshell

We've covered a lot of ground in this chapter, but as you can see, it's all quite simple and logical. I've done my best to turn some complex physiology and nutritional math into a simple series of daily action strategies.

These are the major premises of the high-low nutrition method:

1. Be constantly aware of the importance of a calorie deficit for fat loss.
2. Achieve that deficit easily and automatically by eating primarily low-calorie-density, high-satiety foods.
3. Attain optimum health by eating high-nutrient-density foods.

That's it in a nutshell. It's now time to learn how to maximize your metabolism and burn more calories twenty-four hours a day.

CHAPTER SEVEN

The "E-Max" Fat-Burning Solution

Maximizing Your Metabolism and Burning More Calories Twenty-four Hours a Day

THE most likely environmental factor contributing to the obesity epidemic is a continued decline in daily energy expenditure that has not been matched by an equivalent reduction in energy intake. Increasing physical activity may be the strategy of choice for public health efforts to prevent obesity.

—DR. JAMES HILL, UNIVERSITY OF COLORADO

One of the biggest "food fights" of all time took place recently live on national TV during *Larry King Live*. In one corner sat a best-selling diet book author arguing that exercise was not only unnecessary, he went so far as to say, "Exercise could actually make you fatter." In the other corner was a top celebrity trainer who had helped countless men and women lose up to one hundred pounds or more with vigorous exercise programs combined with a balanced, reduced-calorie diet. She said that "dissing" exercise was doing a

133

massive disservice to the public and was just a convenient way to sell more low-carb diet books. Needless to say, the argument got heated. In the end, I'm not sure that any of the one million viewers were better off after these two duked it out.

The Diet-Versus-Exercise Debate Explained

You would think it's common sense to exercise, but such debates are not unusual today. There are two major reasons for this. The first is that some people really do exercise a lot but still don't lose weight. Clinical researchers have found that a fixed amount of exercise doesn't lead to the same amount of weight loss in all individuals. Initially, this may seem like confirmation that exercise is not effective for weight loss after all or that there's a difference in each person's biological ability to lose fat.

Further studies revealed the truth: when some people started exercising, they ate more. Researchers call them "compensators." Some compensators ate more because exercise increased their physical appetite. In other cases, it was purely psychological. The compensators believed that after hitting the gym and working up a sweat, they deserved to eat more.

The second reason is that conventional aerobic exercise doesn't burn as many calories as most people think. Typically, light to moderate cardio such as brisk walking or jogging burns 5 to 10 calories per minute or less. In a thirty-minute workout, that's only 150 to 300 calories. Some people find that depressing. They thought for sure they were burning 500, 600, even 800 calories. Then they think about the large number of calories in food and imagine how easy it would be to put those 300 calories right back in their mouths at the next meal or snack. All it would take is two ounces of chocolate, two beers, or one slice of pepperoni pizza.

With that logic, they conclude that to get the one- or two-pound weekly weight loss they want, it would be easier to cut food intake by 500 to 1,000 calories per day than to burn that many calories with exercise. In a sense, they're right.

Without reducing food intake, it can be tough to burn enough calories to get a sufficient deficit. On the other hand, to say exercise doesn't work because you overate afterward is ridiculous.

Two Sides to the Fat-Burning Equation

There's only one way to reduce body fat: you must create a calorie deficit. But there are two sides to the fat-burning equation. Instead of thinking about either diet or exercise, the optimal approach is to use both. My goal is to show you how to find the ideal combination between the two.

I've lost track of how many of my clients insisted they could lose weight faster than two pounds a week just by dieting harder, but they never thought through the math. Jennifer, for example, was one of my private coaching clients. She was thirty-six years old, 151 pounds, 28 percent body fat, and only lightly active. This meant her maintenance level was around 2,000 calories per day.

Jennifer was convinced that if she was strict enough with her diet, she could lose three pounds of fat per week or more. "After all," she insisted, "the people in those weight-loss contests and makeover shows on TV are doing it." Only when I crunched the numbers for her did she realize it wasn't realistic.

To get a three-pound weekly weight loss with diet alone would require a 1,500-calorie deficit. That would mean a 500-calorie-per-day starvation diet. If she cut her calories that much, she would be ravenously hungry. She would be cutting her intake of vital nutrients, her energy levels would plummet, and her appetite would increase. She'd also be in danger of losing muscle and eventually gaining back the fat. At the other extreme, if she didn't change her nutrition, she would have to exercise for hours every day to burn 1,500 calories. The math just didn't work.

I advised her instead to set a fat-loss goal of two pounds per week and increase her calorie burning by 500 calories per day, using strength training and any cardio activity of her choosing. With this approach, she was able to raise her metabolic rate to 2,500 calories per day. This allowed her to eat 1,500 calories and still have the deficit she needed to lose two pounds every week. Even if she went over by an extra 250 or even 500 calories some days, she was still in a calorie deficit, and she kept on burning fat.

Controlling calorie intake is important, but calorie cutting alone is not ideal. To burn the maximum amount of fat, boost your metabolism, and build muscle, you need to work more on the calorie-burning side of the equation. I call this approach "e-max," which is simply our shorthand for "maximizing twenty-four-hour energy expenditure." The advantage of e-max is that you don't just lose weight, you get stronger, fitter, and you improve your muscle-to-fat ratio.

The Four Factors of E-Max

In Chapter Six you learned about the selective reduction of calories, which focused your attention where it mattered on the food intake side—on calorie control, not carb control. On the energy expenditure side, the e-max concept again puts your focus where it belongs—on total calories burned, not the type of fuel burned, how it's burned, or when you burn it.

You are going to increase your total calorie expenditure by focusing primarily on two types of formal exercise: weight training and cardio. This chapter will concentrate mainly on the cardio, plus a few other "neat" tricks to get you burning more calories around the clock. Before we get into those details, let's look at the bigger picture by reviewing the four major e-max factors: expenditure, efficiency, enjoyability, and expandability.

1. The Expenditure Factor

If all other factors remain equal, the more energy you use, the more fat you will lose. One roadblock you may have experienced in the past is a fitness myth called the "fat-burning zone." This myth suggests that you should exercise at low intensity to lose body fat. Low-intensity exercise does burn more fat during the workout. The problem is, it doesn't burn as many total calories. When you exercise at a higher intensity, you burn more carbohydrates than fat for fuel during the workout, but you burn far more calories and, therefore, more fat overall. At the end of the day, all the calories you burned might best be considered together as one big pool of energy. The fat-burning zone theory fails to deliver because it doesn't look at the total energy expended. The e-max approach gets you burning as many calories as you can all day long and keeps that up consistently over time.

2. The Efficiency Factor

The most efficient workout is the one that burns the most calories per unit of time. Low-intensity steady-state (LISS) cardio will burn fat just as surely as high-intensity cardio. But low-intensity exercise is less efficient because it burns fewer calories per unit of time. This means that if all else remains equal, using low-intensity cardio will require a greater frequency or duration, or it will take you longer to reach the same goal.

Everyone should be concerned with efficiency to at least some degree, but the more you're pressed for time, the more important efficiency will be for you. You can increase efficiency by gradually progressing into higher-intensity forms of exercise. You could take slow walks for an hour every day, which would go a long way toward your body-fat-reduction goals. But what if you gradually started walking at a faster pace so you burned more calories? What if you did some of your walking up hills? What if you added resistance, like a weighted vest? What if you gradually increased from slow to moderate, then finally to higher-intensity cardio? All physical activity burns calories and anything is better than nothing, but increasing your efficiency is how you get better results for every minute you spend training.

3. The Enjoyability Factor

At the age of forty-two, my friend John transformed himself from what he described as a "240-pound physical mess" with 41 percent body fat, to 175 pounds of muscle with six-pack abs. The most surprising part is, he never did cardio in a gym. John lives in the red, rocky hills of Arizona. In addition to his weight lifting, John mountain biked, sometimes for an hour or two a day. Was he burning a lot of calories? You bet. Was he working hard? I suppose that depends on your definition of work. Sometimes fun hobbies can become your biggest calorie burners. If you can find something that is effective, efficient, and enjoyable, you'll have the best of all worlds.

A program can be highly effective and efficient, but if it doesn't suit your disposition or if it's too extreme to adopt as part of your lifestyle, then it will fail you in the long run. Hard work is always necessary for success, but for some people, the line between work and play is blurred because they enjoy their training so much. In some cases, the enjoyment even turns into passion.

4. The Expandability Factor

Expandability is our e-word to describe the principle of progression. Progression means a workout that may be hard now will eventually get easier as your body adapts and you get in better shape. As your strength, endurance, and fitness levels increase, you need to challenge yourself and gradually expand into more advanced workouts if you want to keep making progress.

All good training programs allow for progression or expansion through as many variables as possible. To break a progress plateau or accelerate your results, you can progressively increase the intensity, frequency, or duration of your workouts because total calories burned will be a product of these three variables. It's important, of course, to start at your own level and build up slowly. As a beginner, it's tempting to admire the body of an athlete or fitness model and copy their workout with no regard to your own capacity. Unfortunately, that kind of overenthusiasm could lead to compliance problems or even injury.

The Critical Factor

The most critical of the four factors is total daily energy expenditure. The simple proven fact of body-fat reduction is that if all else remains equal, and you burn more calories, you'll lose more body fat. If you keep asking yourself, "How do I burn more calories?" you'll be headed down the right path every time. If you're busy, then you must ask, "How do I burn more calories in less time?" If you've had problems with compliance, then you ask, "How do I burn more calories and have fun doing it so it doesn't seem like work?"

The Six Points of Energy Expenditure

So, how do you burn more calories? Obviously, you exercise more, but did you know that there are a total of six ways to increase your energy expenditure? Even better news is that you can influence every one of them, sometimes in a big way.

The key to increasing your metabolism and burning more calories is to break down your total daily energy expenditure into each of its individual parts, and then rev up each area to the highest degree possible. Let's take a look at each one.

1. Resting Metabolic Rate (RMR)

Resting metabolic rate, or RMR, is the amount of energy you use just for essential body functions. Your RMR is the largest component of your daily energy expenditure, representing 60–75 percent of the total calories you burn every day. If you could increase the amount of calories you burned at rest, this would have a huge impact on your body fat levels over time.

The long-term effect of cardio on RMR is still being researched, but there are two things we know for sure: first, you can temporarily elevate your RMR with intense cardio, as well as strength training. Second, your RMR is directly related to the amount of muscle you have. If you lose muscle from extreme dieting, then your RMR will decrease. If you gain muscle from supportive nutrition and weight training, then your RMR will increase.

2. Weight Training

Many people avoid weight training because they believe it has nothing to do with fat loss. It does. Many women avoid weight training because they think it will make them bulky. It doesn't. Weight training has the potential to burn as many calories as cardio, while simultaneously revving up two other points of energy expenditure: resting metabolic rate (through increased lean body mass) and post-workout metabolic rate.

Effective weight training can burn 7 to 9 calories per minute and more, even when you count the rest intervals. Weight training is not simply for building muscle and getting stronger. Always focus on total calories burned and recognize the impact of weight training on lean muscle. Then you'll realize that weight training may be the most important but underappreciated and neglected type of exercise for burning body fat.

3. Cardio Training

Cardio training is one of the best ways to burn calories and reduce your body fat. The number of calories you burn during cardio varies based on intensity, duration, and frequency. As long as your food intake stays the same, there will be a direct relationship between the volume of cardio you do and the amount of fat you will lose.

Steady cardio sessions of approximately forty-five minutes at moderate intensities or twenty- to thirty-minute sessions at high intensities can burn very significant amounts of energy. If the intensity is high enough, some calories are burned after the workout, as well as from increased postexercise metabolism. But in most cases, the majority of the calories are burned during the exercise session itself.

4. Excess Postexercise Oxygen Consumption (EPOC)

After intense or prolonged exercise, your metabolism stays elevated for twelve to twenty-four hours, and in extreme cases, for up to forty-eight hours. Exercise physiologists call this excess postexercise oxygen consumption (EPOC). Some trainers call it the afterburn effect.

The amount of extra calories burned from EPOC is related to intensity and duration, but intensity is the critical factor. Increases in duration produce a linear increase in EPOC, while increases in intensity produce an exponential increase in EPOC. The downside is that EPOC only kicks in after very intense exercise, such as high-intensity interval training (HIIT). Beginners and overweight people usually can't safely generate the kind of intensity needed to get a significant afterburn, so they often have to depend on longer, less-intense sessions to get the same results.

5. Thermic Effect of Food (TEF)

Every time you eat a meal, your metabolic rate increases due to the energy cost of digestion. This is known as the thermic effect of food (TEF) and it accounts for about 10 percent of your energy expenditure. As you learned in Chapter Six, one way you can increase TEF is by eating more highly thermic foods. Shifting to a higher percentage of lean protein can increase TEF. Although the difference is small, it's enough to explain why a high-protein diet can produce a slightly greater weight loss than the same amount of calories at a lower intake of protein. Protein is also a great appetite suppressant. When you're in a calorie deficit, eating enough protein helps spare your muscle. Research has shown that even the substitution of one serving of saturated fat or refined carbs for one serving of lean protein is enough to make a difference in body composition.

6. Nonexercise Activity Thermogenesis (NEAT)

As the name implies, NEAT is all your physical activity throughout the day, outside of formal exercise or sports. This includes all the calories you burn from activity at work, as well as standing, pacing, walking, dancing, shopping, gardening, housework, and even things like talking, chewing, changing posture, and fidgeting (which obviously don't burn many calories, but they do require energy).

Although it may appear insignificant, if you manipulate your NEAT in minor ways throughout the day, the results can add up in a big way over the long term.

The Body Fat Solution Cardio Rx: What Kind, How Long, How Often, How Hard, and Other Frequently Asked Questions About Fat-Burning Exercise

Keeping the four e-max factors and the six points of energy expenditure in mind will make all your training decisions easy. You'll never have a doubt about whether you're on the right track. The best part is, this fat-burning exercise formula is a flexible and adaptable set of guidelines rather than one strict prescription. Instead of getting a canned workout program, the Body Fat Solution cardio prescription teaches you universal principles. This lets you write your own personal fat-burning program that suits your schedule and lifestyle no matter what level you're starting from today.

What Kind?

When most people think of fat-burning exercise, they think of aerobics. Unfortunately, the word "aerobics" can carry a lot of emotional baggage, especially for "macho" guys. Thinking in terms of aerobics also tends to restrict you to a fairly narrow list of choices. Most people stereotype aerobics as a group step class, jogging for miles, or long sessions of cardio on the elliptical machine or bike. Aerobics does have a scientific definition, but for practical purposes we're not going to worry about that. Our definition of fat-burning exercise is much more flexible. We call it cardio. In the Body Fat Solution program, cardio includes any physical activity that increases your breathing and heart rate high enough and long enough to burn a lot of calories. Generally speaking, these are exercises that use large muscle groups, namely your legs or your arms and legs together, and they elevate your breathing and heart rate. They can be done continuously at a steady pace for a long period, or in intermittent bouts at a higher intensity separated by bouts of rest or lower-intensity work.

This definition of cardio leaves you almost spoiled for choice and gives you more room to work the enjoyability factor into the equation. Here are some suggestions:

- walking/hiking
- jogging/running
- elliptical/cross-trainer machine
- stair-climbing
- cycling
- rowing
- swimming/water exercise
- cross-country skiing
- high-energy-cost group exercise classes (or videos)
- bodyweight exercises or calisthenics
- high-energy-cost sports (boxing, basketball, tennis, racquetball, soccer)

How Long?

Another simple way to burn more calories is to train longer. If you double your duration at the same intensity, you will double your energy expenditure and double your fat loss, assuming your food intake remains the same. Of course, there are drawbacks to doing longer cardio sessions. One is the potential for overuse injury if your training volume gets too high. Most people don't want to spend an hour or two in the gym every day. The solution for a time-restricted situation is to find an efficient balance between reducing calories and increasing activity and do just as much cardio as it takes to reach your weekly goals.

A problem with prescribing cardio workouts by time alone is that it fails to take intensity into account. It's important to think about the inverse relationship between intensity and duration and how that affects your total calorie expenditure and time required to exercise. If you exercise with high intensity, your optimal duration could be as little as twenty to thirty minutes per session. If you exercise with moderate intensity, your optimal duration is probably in the thirty-to forty-five-minute range. If you exercise with low intensity, your optimal duration is probably closer to forty-five to sixty minutes. Each of these workouts could burn a similar amount of calories due to the different intensity levels.

When you're first starting out, you'll need to begin with low- to moderate-intensity training and build up your duration gradually until you reach these optimal time frames. If the best you can manage is ten minutes on your first workout, that's great. Gradually increase your duration to the optimal times as your fitness level increases.

How Often?

Exercise physiologists and weight-loss experts have deduced that there's a minimum threshold of cardio necessary *if you want to optimize your rate of fat loss.* That amount is usually three days per week at thirty minutes with sufficient intensity to burn at least 300 calories a session. Three days per week of cardio in conjunction with three days per week of strength training and a conservative food reduction is a great way to get started. We're going to call that our training "baseline."

Once you've established your baseline, if you want to burn more calories, accelerate your results, or break a fat-loss plateau, you can increase your cardio frequency to four to six days per week, if time permits. There's no reason not to exercise seven days a week if you choose, but most people find that leaving one day of complete rest gives them a nicer balance in life and leads to better long-term compliance.

If you decide to increase your training frequency beyond three days per week, it's usually smart to limit the higher-intensity forms of cardio to three days a week. Use lower or moderate cardio on the other days to prevent injury, over-training, or mental burnout.

How Hard?

Intensity refers to how hard you work in terms of metabolic cost or oxygen consumed. Intensity is relative. If you're a sedentary beginner, walking up one flight of stairs can leave you gasping for air with your heart pounding, so that would be intense, relatively speaking. If you're highly conditioned, a 10k run could be a breeze.

The traditional way to measure exercise intensity is with heart rate. The classic formula for estimated maximal heart rate is 220 minus your age. The optimal training zone for cardiorespiratory fitness benefits and a significant calorie burn is 70–85 percent of maximal heart rate. As a general rule, the higher your heart rate during exercise, the harder you're working and the more energy you're expending.

Prescribing workouts by heart rate is not a perfect science, but it's valuable and useful to measure your heart rate while you work out, if not as a target, then at least as a reference point and accountability tool. You can do this with a heart rate monitor or by taking a ten-second pulse count at your neck or wrist and multiplying by six.

An alternative to target heart rate is to use the Borg rating of perceived exertion (RPE). As you might guess, it was invented by a guy named Borg, and although it may seem too simplistic to be accurate, RPE gives you an estimate that

RATING OF PERCEIVED EXERTION (RPE)

Score	Traditional Borg Scale	Type of Cardio/Activity	Abbreviation
0	Nothing at all	Sitting or lying in bed	BMR
1	Very weak	Nonexercise work or activity	NEAT
2	Weak	Nonexercise work or activity	NEAT
3	Moderate	Low-intensity steady-state	LISS
4	Somewhat strong	Low-intensity steady-state	LISS
5	Strong	Moderate-intensity steady-state	MISS
6		Moderate-intensity steady-state	MISS
7	Very strong	Intense steady-state	HISS
8		Intense long-interval	HIIT
9		Intense short-interval	HIIT
10	Very, very strong	All-out maximum sprint	HIIT

correlates remarkably well to actual intensity and heart rate. It's also very practical because most people find it easy to rate things from 1 to 10.

Never start with high-intensity training. Start slowly at an intensity you're comfortable with and build up gradually as you become more fit. If you're a beginner, I recommend you build an aerobic base for about one month with LISS cardio before attempting any kind of higher-intensity training.

High-Intensity Interval Training (HIIT)

If you want to burn the most calories possible, the way to do it is to combine high intensity and long duration. The problem, of course, is that intensity and duration are inversely related, or as they say, "You can't sprint through a marathon." In fact, you can't even sprint for ten minutes. An all-out sprint will last only seconds and an 85–90 percent–effort sprint may last only a minute or two. There is a way, however, to combine high intensity and longer duration, and that is called interval training.

An interval workout consists of a short burst of high-intensity work followed by lower-intensity recovery periods. Then you repeat for a prescribed number of rounds. Interval training can be done with very intense bursts as brief as 15 to 30 seconds, or with longer high-intensity intervals of 60 to 120 seconds. If work intervals are too short, the workout may become impractical, especially on cardio machines where you have to change the speed, incline, or resistance. If work intervals are too long, then they're no longer true high-intensity intervals, they're just aerobic intervals. Most interval training workouts call for somewhere between six and twelve rounds (sometimes more when very short intervals are used).

You can do interval training on any cardio machine, such as a bike or treadmill, or you could walk, jog, or run outdoors up flat surfaces, up hills, or up stadium stairs. There are many variations and there's really no right or wrong way. For body-fat reduction, you can finish an effective interval workout in as little as twenty to twenty-five minutes. For health and cardiorespiratory fitness, even shorter interval workouts have proven benefits.

Beginner Interval Workout (4 rounds @ 1:2 work/recovery ratio)—Month 1

Warm up for five minutes steady state at a low RPE.

Work interval: perform one minute of moderately intense work at 7 to 8 RPE.

Recovery interval: perform two minutes of steady-state pace at 3 to 4 RPE.

Repeat for four more work intervals.

Cool down for five minutes at a low RPE.

Total workout time: 22 minutes.

Intermediate Interval Workout (6 rounds @ 1:1 work/recovery ratio)—Month 2

Warm up for five minutes steady state at a low RPE.

Work interval: perform one minute of intense work at 8 to 9 RPE.

Recovery interval: perform one minute of steady-state pace at 3 to 4 RPE.

Repeat for six to eight work intervals

Cool down for five minutes at a low RPE.

Total workout time: 22 to 26 minutes.

Advanced Interval Workout (8 to 10 rounds @ 1:1 work/recovery ratio)—Month 3 and Beyond

Warm up for five minutes steady state at a low RPE.

Work interval: perform one minute of very intense work at 9 to 10 RPE.

Recovery interval: perform one minute of steady-state pace at 3 to 4 RPE.

Repeat for eight to ten work intervals.

Cool down for five minutes at a low RPE.

Total workout time: 26 to 30 minutes.

Cruise Control Cardio (HISS)

Another type of cardio that burns a very large amount of calories is steady-state training pinned at the highest intensity you can maintain for any given duration. I call this "cruise control" cardio because it's similar to what you probably do when driving on the highway. You usually set your cruise control at or just below the posted speed limit. At that speed, you'd get to your destination the fastest, because if you were to go any faster, you would get pulled over by your friendly state trooper and have to stop, thereby defeating the purpose of going faster in the first place.

Cruise control cardio recognizes that the total amount of calories you burn will be a product of intensity times duration. It's the opposite of the slow-go "fat-burning zone" mentality. However much time you have—fifteen minutes, thirty minutes, forty-five minutes, whatever—the more intensely you work during that period, the more energy you'll expend and the more fat you'll burn. It's that simple. For this reason, another name for this is "highest-intensity steady-state," or HISS, cardio.

Some people believe steady-state cardio is always low in intensity. But steady-state workouts can and should be challenging too. The main point is that if you push yourself a little bit harder, you can always burn more calories and get to your destination faster.

Does It Matter What You Burn? The Fat-Burning Zone Debunked

The biggest myth about cardio is the belief that you must exercise aerobically at a slower pace to burn body fat, and if you burn sugar you will not lose body fat. This is also known as the fat-burning zone myth (not to be confused with a target heart rate, which is prescribed for cardiovascular fitness purposes).

The fat-burning zone theory is based on substrate utilization, which means the type of fuel you burn during a workout. During low-intensity exercise, you burn a greater proportion of fuel from fat. On this basis, some people figure that low-intensity exercise burns more body fat over time. There are serious flaws in this thinking. First is that low-intensity exercise doesn't burn very many calories. Second, not only does higher-intensity exercise burn more total calories, it can easily burn as many calories from fat during the workout as low-intensity cardio, and sometimes more. Here's an example:

Low-Intensity Exercise—30 Minutes

Fuel mix: 50% fat, 50% carbs

Carbs burned: 110 calories

Fat burned: 110 calories

Total calories burned: 220

High-Intensity Exercise—30 Minutes

Fuel mix: 33% fat, 67% carbs

Carbs burned: 222 calories

Fat burned: 110 calories

Total calories burned: 332

Third, focusing only on what fuel gets burned during the workout is only part of the picture. What about the other twenty-three hours of the day? Fat oxidation does matter, but if you burn more carbohydrates during your workout, your body compensates over twenty-four hours and burns more fat later in the day, so it appears to be a wash. The focus of e-max is on how many total calories you burn every twenty-four hours, not just what you burn during the workout.

Moderate exercise burns more calories than light exercise. Intense exercise burns more calories than moderate exercise. Work harder, burn more calories, lose more fat. If you're still not convinced that the fat-burning zone is useless, then look at it this way: sitting on your couch is a low-intensity (fat-burning) activity. Why not sit on your couch all day long? Because couch sitting only burns about one calorie per minute.

Do You Have to Do High-Intensity Exercise?

With all this talk about training intensely, you might be concerned or intimidated, especially if you're older, overweight, or you've never worked out before.

Don't worry. You don't have to do high-intensity exercise. In fact, high-intensity exercise can be dangerous if you've been inactive, if you don't have your doctor's approval for vigorous exercise, if you're obese, or if you're susceptible to orthopedic stress or joint problems. For many people who are overweight, LISS cardio such as walking is the single best choice.

You need to decide if high-intensity exercise is appropriate for you, and that includes the enjoyability factor. If you can't tolerate intense exercise physically or psychologically, then don't do it. Low- and moderate-intensity exercise is not ineffective, it simply takes a little more time or volume to burn the same amount of fat. You can also get significant health benefits even with small amounts of light or moderate exercise. Remember, health must go high on your values list and your outcome is to be lean and healthy, not one or the other.

Do You Have to Exercise in One Long Session, or Can You Break It Up?

Years ago, most fitness experts believed that you had to exercise for at least twenty minutes in one long session before you started to burn fat. Recent research has found that long continuous sessions are not a necessity and that cumulative time is what matters. If you prefer to break up your cardio training into three ten-minute sessions or two fifteen-minute sessions instead of one thirty-minute session, your results will be similar either way. You might even get better results with two shorter sessions because your metabolism could be stimulated with two post-workout afterburn effects.

Japanese researchers at the University of Tokyo recently compared a single long bout of exercise with repeated bouts at an equivalent intensity and duration. They found that the repeated bouts actually induced greater fat metabolism. More research is needed to confirm whether short multiple bouts give you any major advantage over the long term, so for now the best choice is probably the option that fits into your lifestyle most easily.

Do You Need to Count How Many Calories You Burn?

Throughout this chapter, I've emphasized the importance of burning calories, so you may be wondering if you need to figure out how many calories you burn during each workout. While it's a great idea to journal and quantify as many things as possible, it's not necessary to count calories burned during your workouts. It's also unrealistic for most people to manually add up the calories you burn during each activity throughout the day. As with caloric intake from food, you only need to understand the concept of calorie expenditure from exercise and be able to apply it on a practical level to make it work for you.

If you're the detail-oriented analytical type or if you're a gadget geek, then by all means, use tools such as electronic calorie counters, heart rate monitors, and associated software to tally up your energy expended. It could be a real eye-opener. But consider it optional. The way to tell if you're burning enough calories is to look at your results. Is your body fat decreasing or not? If not, then you're in energy balance and you need to reestablish an energy deficit using one side of the equation or the other, eat less or burn more.

Does It Matter When You Burn the Calories?

Many people believe that doing cardio first thing in the morning before breakfast improves results because fat oxidation during cardio is increased when you're in the fasted state. How much this affects total fat loss over twenty-four hours and extended periods is still being debated. At best, the time of day you work out and whether it is done fasted is secondary to how many total calories you burn. Schedule your workouts for the time that you're most likely to enjoy it and stick with it. It may also be beneficial to train at the same time every day so you take advantage of the power of habit. One more important tip about timing: I recommend you don't perform your cardio before weight training because that would leave you fatigued, and your weight training would probably suffer.

NEAT Ways to Burn More Fat

Researchers say that NEAT, which is all the calories you burn every day outside your formal exercise sessions, is the reason there's so much difference between individuals in total daily calorie expenditure. Dr. James Levine, an endocrinologist and the top researcher in the field says, "Obese people are profoundly more sedentary than lean people. They move 2.5 hours less per day than lean people, which means they burn roughly 350 fewer calories per day."

For most people, NEAT accounts for about 30 percent of physical activity calories spent daily, but NEAT can run as low as 15 percent in sedentary individuals and as high as 50 percent in highly active individuals. Walking contributes to the majority of NEAT. Obviously, the type of work you do is a major influence on NEAT. If you work at a desk all day long and hardly get up, your NEAT level is low. If you deliver mail, or work any other type of physical job, your NEAT can be quite high.

The fact that most people sit all day long and surf the Web, watch TV, and play video games is not a minor factor in the obesity problem. We have become a desk-bound, technology-based society. One hundred fifty years ago, 90 percent of the world's population worked in agriculture or did some type of physical labor to earn a living. "The human body evolved over a million years, but the car-computer-chair-elevator-television-based world has evolved in less than a century," says Dr. Levine, "so you're imposing a massive environmental change on a very old biology. No wonder it all goes haywire."

Short of changing your job from desk jockey to lumberjack, you may be thinking that NEAT is too trivial to amount to anything. If you looked at it one activity at a time, you'd probably be right. However, when you look at it from the long-term perspective, and when you make small changes in daily activities that become a habitual part of your lifestyle, it accumulates over the months and years.

You can implement a NEAT strategy by thinking about simple ways you can become more active and including them in your daily behavioral goals. Here are some ideas:

- Take the stairs instead of the elevator.
- Stand or pace more instead of sitting.
- Get a desk treadmill or mini-stepper.
- Get out of your chair and walk around, stretch, or do some body weight exercises on the hour, every hour while working at your desk.
- Do not use labor-saving devices all the time (riding mowers, leaf blowers, snowblowers, golf carts, and so on).
- Do some of your own housework or yard work.
- For short local trips and errands, walk instead of taking a cab or driving.
- Look for other opportunities to walk more (walk your dog, for example).
- Spend less leisure time watching TV, surfing the Internet, or playing video games, and more time engaging in physical recreation, sports, boating, cycling, hiking, and so forth.
- Watch less TV, unless you're watching it on a treadmill or stationary bike.
- If you have kids, get as much physical activity with them as possible.
- Be aware of seasonal variations, especially if you live somewhere with harsh winters. The difference between summer and winter activity can vary twofold. (It's not just holiday food that causes winter weight gain.)

Out of all these tips, do your best to spend less time in a chair and more time walking. You may even want to invest in a pedometer, which will tally up your steps every day. A 2006 study published in the *American Journal of Health Promotion* found that in previously sedentary overweight adults, subjects who met a ten-thousand-steps-per-day goal saw large improvements in body composition. Those who missed their goal did not.

Also consider the older-order Amish culture, where modern labor-saving technology has not been fully adopted. Among these Amish, the obesity rate is only 4 percent, compared to 30 percent in the United States overall. A pedometer study published in *Medicine and Science in Sports and Exercise* reported that Amish men walked an average of 18,425 steps per day and women 14,196 steps. The average American logs in about five thousand steps a day. That's a difference of four hundred to six hundred calories per day, which gives us a good approximation of how physical activity has changed as technology has advanced over the past century. Most interesting of all, the diet of the Amish was not low in carbs or low in calories—it included meat, eggs, gravy, potatoes, bread, and even pies and cakes. The Amish stayed trim by balancing their food intake with high activity.

There's a common misconception among some trainers and serious fitness enthusiasts that if exercise isn't high in intensity, then it's ineffective. Research studies like these prove that this is not true at all and that walking (low-intensity cardio) is an effective way to beat body fat. It may not get the job done as quickly, but it gets it done just the same. Anything is better than sitting all day long.

Do Whatever You Can . . . Right Now

Over the years, I've received thousands of testimonials, letters, and success story e-mails. I received one recently that I will never forget. The message said:

> TOM, I'M THIRTY-SEVEN YEARS OLD and have been paralyzed from the neck down for more than eleven years. Due to my level of inactivity and my total lack of understanding of physiology and nutrition, my eating habits and body fat fluctuated significantly and had been a constant source of frustration. I can't do much on the exercise front, as you can imagine, but using your information on calories and the best foods to eat, I was able to slim down significantly. I'm not sure how many pounds I lost, as I am unable to be weighed, but yesterday evening, my doctor came over for dinner and immediately said I was looking especially slim and well. Much appreciated and many thanks.
>
> JOEL

I was very moved after I read this, but this also teaches every one of us an important practical lesson: exercise is not a requirement for weight loss. The only absolute necessity is a caloric deficit. I'm not backpedaling and suggesting that you don't exercise. Quite the opposite—I'm a huge advocate of exercise and lots of it. The reason I'm concluding with this story is because if we don't acknowledge that a calorie deficit is the necessity, and not the type of exercise program, then we might lose sight of the true core of the solution and some folks who are not fully mobile might get discouraged and not even try.

Many people believe that if they can't do it all—full-out exercise and diet— they might as well do nothing. My advice: "Do what you can, with what you have, wherever you are, right now," as Theodore Roosevelt once said. If you can't do a certain type of exercise, do something else. If you can't do much now, then start slowly and add more later. If you can't exercise at all, simply restrict your food intake in a sensible manner. It may not be the optimal approach, but you'll lose weight just the same. If you adopt this can-do attitude, then you can begin with the hope, knowledge, and confidence that you can achieve your ideal weight no matter what your present circumstances.

The "Lean Muscle" Training Solution

Reshaping Your Body and Getting Leaner with Weight Training

> **IF YOU** do only cardio and no strength training, you can expect to lose strength, gain fat, struggle with lower-back pain, and eventually become more reliant on others for physical tasks. Balance the right types of cardio with the right type of strength training and you can build and preserve muscle as you age and remain lean, strong, and injury free.
>
> —DR. JOHN BERARDI, PH.D., EXERCISE PHYSIOLOGY AND NUTRITIONAL BIOCHEMISTRY

Linda just didn't get it. The idea that weight lifting would help her get slimmer didn't compute. Like so many of my new clients, she thought that weight lifting was anaerobic, which means it burns carbs as the primary fuel source. "If it doesn't burn fat," she asked, "then why should I bother to lift weights? And besides," she concluded," I don't want to get bulky, I just want to be thin."

After I let out a big sigh, I prepared to step onto my soapbox for what must

157

have been the two thousandth presentation of my "Why weight training is the key to a lean, hot body" lecture. Yes, the same one I'm about to give you. Why should you listen? Ask Linda. When she first came to see me, she weighed a mushy 178 pounds. When she finished the program, she weighed a solid 138 pounds with a totally new body shape.

More important, she didn't merely lose weight, her body composition improved. This means she burned the fat and actually gained lean body mass in the process. And no, that doesn't mean she gained muscular bulk. She looks lean, strong, healthy, and athletic. That's the kind of body you get from weight training. It's a completely different look from what you'd get from losing weight without training.

Why Weight Training Must Be Your Top Priority

Weight training will make you stronger and more muscular. But there's more to it than that. When you add dedicated weight training to your fitness regime, while fueling yourself properly with nutrient-dense, natural food, you increase your calorie expenditure and boost your metabolism. You also create a hormonal environment that tells your body to hold on to lean tissue while you're burning off fat.

Previously, we established that burning fat requires a calorie deficit. You can achieve a calorie deficit by reducing your food intake alone, if need be, but that's not the best approach. Adding exercise makes it easier to achieve a substantial deficit and reach your fat-burning goals faster. If you created your caloric deficit with cardio alone, however, you'd have a difficult time maintaining your lean body mass during the deficit.

Most people don't think about weight training in a weight-loss program, or they don't consider it a priority. It seems incomprehensible, but it's not uncommon for weight-loss centers to advise their clients not to lift weights. Their ulterior motive? The center has promised that their client will lose a certain amount of weight by following their program, but they know adding muscle can slow down weight loss on the scale.

Do you know how hard it is to convince scale-focused folks that it's okay to gain weight as long as it's muscle? It's darn near impossible. So, they cop out and discourage weight training. The truth is, there's no substitute for weight training. In case you're still not sold yet, here are six reasons to reconsider:

1. Weight training is the best way to maintain your muscle in a calorie deficit

Anytime you reduce your calories, you run the risk of losing lean body mass along with the fat. The more you cut calories and the longer you stay on a reduced-calorie diet, the greater the risk. Without weight training, your body can easily get a large proportion of its energy needs by cannibalizing muscle. Adding resistance training, with weights or body-weight resistance, helps you maintain your muscle when your calories are low.

2. Weight training burns calories and increases fat loss

Weight training can also contribute in a major way to your total daily energy expenditure while building muscle at the same time. Give me a few good sets of squats, lunges, and dead lifts and I can guarantee you'll have burned at least as many if not more calories than you would have in the same time spent on a cardio machine.

3. Weight training increases your metabolism

Weight training is not only a superb calorie burner, it's also a great metabolism booster. Weight training creates microtrauma to the muscle fibers, which must be repaired during the recovery period between workouts. This process is metabolically costly because it takes a lot of energy to repair damaged muscle and synthesize new lean tissue. Research has also demonstrated that weight training can actually stimulate a greater postexercise metabolism-boosting effect than cardio.

4. Weight training improves your health

There's a huge misconception that only aerobic exercise is good for your heart and overall health. Physicians, public health officials, and exercise organizations have finally started coming around. Almost all of them now recommend weight training for heart health, improved blood cholesterol profiles, strengthened bone density, increased insulin sensitivity, and other health benefits.

5. Weight training is the chisel you use to sculpt and shape your body

Some fitness experts say you can't "shape" a muscle. Naturally, you can't change the origins and insertions of your muscles or your overall bone structure, but you can totally reshape your body with resistance training. With diet alone, you may end up nothing more than a smaller version of your old self. With training, you can chisel away at unwanted fat and slap on muscle exactly where you want it, in the exact amount you want. Think of your body as a living, breathing sculpture—a work of art always in progress—and weight training is your primary tool.

6. Weight training helps reverse the aging process

As you get older and become more concerned about looking and feeling youthful, you have a couple of choices. You could go to an antiaging clinic, get expensive prescriptions for drugs and hormones, slog down all kinds of goop, swallow fifty different supplement pills a day, and hope that one of these things will be the fountain of youth. Or, you could change your attitudes and beliefs by following the ten Body Fat Solution nutrition rules and lift weights.

People who don't maintain their lean body mass through strength training will lose up to 40 percent of their muscle by age sixty-five. This progressive muscle loss with age is so insidious it has been given a scientific name: sarcopenia. Although many people accept this deterioration as unavoidable, most sedentary people experience accelerated pathological aging, not normal aging. When it comes to muscles, "use it or lose it" is literally true. When you understand this, you realize that weight training is as close to the fountain of youth as you will ever get.

Supersets: An Ideal Choice for Effective, Time-Efficient Fat-Loss Training

Since we've now agreed that weight training gets you leaner, stronger, biologically younger, and makes you look good naked, the next question is, what kind of training program should you follow? There are so many programs these days it seems almost impossible to choose. But when it comes to fat loss, one style of weight training is clearly head and shoulders above the rest. The technique is called supersetting, and it's the foundation of the Body Fat Solution training program.

Conventional strength training is usually done using straight sets. One repetition, or rep, is each time you lift and lower a weight. A straight set consists of a series of nonstop repetitions, usually somewhere between five and fifteen, followed by a brief rest interval of about a minute or two. A superset is where you perform two exercises in a row with no rest in between them.

Supersetting may be superior for fat-burning workouts because you can perform more work in less time. The amount of work you perform in a given time is known as density. Increasing density by using supersets places a greater overload on your muscles and also burns more calories in less time. While not as effective for strength development as straight sets, supersets don't compromise your strength or muscular development substantially, the way that long circuits do.

The effect of supersets on your body is more metabolic in nature, which means that your metabolism and fat-burning hormones are stimulated more with superset training than conventional training with long breaks between sets. Supersets also save you time, and the workouts are much more engaging—a huge plus if you get bored sitting around between sets.

The Benefits of Full-Body Workouts

If your primary goal is fat loss and your time is limited, then full-body workouts with supersets will always be one of your best choices, even after you pass beyond the beginner stage. Full-body workouts are not without downsides, though, which is why many people move to split routines. The good news is, there is a way to combine the best features of full-body and split-training schedules.

Semi-full-body split training is a system popularized by Australian strength coach Ian King. It's a great way to get all the benefits of full-body training without the drawbacks. Using the same exercises performed three days per week assumes your muscles will recover fully with just forty-eight hours between workouts. Sometimes that's not enough time. Semi-full-body split training bypasses this problem because you continue training your full body three days per week, but you change the exercises and movement patterns every other workout.

For example, on Monday you do squats, where the primary emphasis is on the quadriceps muscle group. On Wednesday, you train your lower body again, but instead of squats you do Romanian dead lifts, where the primary emphasis is on the hip and hamstring muscle groups. This way, you still train your lower body every other day, and you still train your entire body every workout, but there are at least ninety-six hours between workouts for each exercise or movement pattern.

Another outstanding feature of this three-day, full-body schedule is that it's a template you can use in the future, even after you finish the two-phase training program in this chapter. You keep the semi-full-body split, stay on the same weekly schedule, and simply plug in new exercises as you learn them. Last but not least, this type of training split helps alleviate the potential boredom that may arise from repeating the same workout for weeks on end.

Dumbbells Are Not for Dummies

The Body Fat Solution program is designed to fit the lifestyles of millions of busy people. For this reason, it is essential that the workout can be done in the privacy of your own home with minimal equipment. That's why you can perform all the exercises with dumbbells or no equipment at all (body weight). If you own a home gym or you train in a public gym, that's even better because you'll have more exercises to choose from.

For home training, there's one piece of equipment that stands above them all. If you're thinking of one of those high-tech contraptions you see on late-night infomercials, think again. The ultimate in home training is the humble dumbbell.

You can start with as few as two or three pairs of dumbbells, which you'll need because the larger muscles such as legs will be much stronger than the smaller arm muscles. As your strength increases, you can progress by adding heavier dumbbells. Of course, that can take up a lot of space and get expensive after a while, so an alternative to solid, fixed-weight dumbbells are free-weight adjustable dumbbells. These consist of dumbbell handles to which you add weight plates and then secure the plates with collars.

A third option that's even more convenient and time-saving is selectorized dumbbells. Three of the better known brands are PowerBlocks, SelectTech by Bowflex, and Ironmaster Quick-Lock dumbbells. These are ingenious little inventions. They save space, time, and money. Literally by pulling a pin or turning a dial, you can change the resistance, which does away with a whole rack of solid dumbbells. If there's any downside, it's that some selectorized dumbbells are not conventionally shaped and have a slightly awkward feel or bulkiness to them, but most people say they get used to it.

Why else should you use dumbbells? Let me count the ways:

- Dumbbells can be used for thousands of exercises.
- Dumbbells can be used for more than twice as many exercises as barbells because you can do unilateral exercises (one arm or leg at a time).
- Dumbbells save you money because they can replace expensive machines or a gym membership.
- Dumbbells save space because they replace bulky weight-training machines.
- Dumbbells provide balanced muscular development because each side of your body must work equally.
- Dumbbells help create a strong and stable core.

- Dumbbells require more balance and activate the neuromuscular system and stabilizer muscles far more than machines and even more than barbells.
- Dumbbells do not lock you into a fixed movement pattern the way machines do, which means the movement is more natural, functional, and less likely to result in injuries.
- Dumbbells are safer than barbells in the event that you have to drop a weight or if you train without a spotter.

The Benefits of Body-Weight Training

There's one more amazing piece of equipment you need to learn how to use: your own body. When you hear the terms "weight training," "resistance training," or "strength training," you may immediately think of barbells, dumbbells, and machines. But remember, your body is a weight. When you do a push-up, you're performing the same movement pattern as a bench press; you're simply using your body as resistance instead of barbells or dumbbells.

Anyone can become fit, burn calories, and even build muscle with body-weight exercises. However, once you can do body-weight exercises for high repetitions with good form, then it makes sense to increase the load and move into free-weight training if you want further improvements in muscle and strength development. One of the greatest advantages of learning body-weight exercises is that you can get a workout at home and in hotel rooms when you're traveling. Quite possibly the single best choice for home strength training is a workout that combines body-weight exercises with dumbbells.

Progressive Overload and Adaptation

When your body is exposed to new physical stress, it first goes through a shock or alarm phase, as the stressor represents a disruption to your body. Your body then moves into an adaptation phase. When muscle fibers are taxed with work they've never done before, they adapt by growing stronger and larger in order to handle that stress in the future.

Training, therefore, is a positive form of stress, provided you don't overdo it and you allow yourself enough time to recover from each workout. If you push too hard, too long, or too often, then instead of adapting in a positive fashion, you pass into an exhaustion phase and begin to see negative physical symptoms. You feel tired, sore, and achy. Your sleep is disrupted, your strength and lean body mass actually decrease, and you may begin to lose your enthusiasm for training. This means you've applied too much stress and not enough recovery.

Understanding the stress response is one of the keys to fitness training success, especially strength training. Once your body has adapted to a workout, if you repeat the same workout, there will no longer be a shock or alarm phase. It's old news. If your muscles could talk, they'd say, "Did that, done that, been there." By repeating a previous workout, you may maintain your level of strength and fitness, but you don't improve it. If you do what you always did, you'll get what you always got. The secret to continuous progress is progressive overload.

You must challenge yourself to go one small step beyond what you've achieved in past workouts, while being sure to allow adequate recovery between the workouts. Most people think of progression only in terms of lifting more weight. However, progressive overload can also come in the form of doing more repetitions, increasing the work performed per unit of time, using advanced intensity techniques, changing the exercises, changing the combinations of exercises, or making your body do some type of physical work it has never done before.

Of course, it's difficult if not impossible to improve your performance and break personal records at every workout indefinitely. But over time, an upward trend of continuous improvement in workout performance should always be your goal.

How to Choose the Best Exercises

There are thousands of exercises you can choose from. As your training experience grows, it pays to learn and use as many exercise variations as possible. That keeps your body stimulated and prevents you from getting bored. However, most exercises are simply variations on a few basic movement patterns. The most effective and time-efficient workouts always revolve around the basics.

The basic exercises that give you the most benefit are the ones that emphasize the major movement patterns, recruit the most muscle mass, involve multiple joints, and require a lot of energy to perform. The squat, for example, involves the hip and knee joints, recruits a huge area of muscle mass, and expends an enormous amount of energy. By contrast, the leg extension machine uses only the knee joint, it primarily isolates the quadriceps group, and does not burn nearly the amount of energy as the squat. That makes the squat and its variations optimal for fat-loss programs and an obvious first choice. Other beneficial exercises include lunges, rows, pulling movements, pressing movements, and core activation exercises.

This doesn't mean you should never do isolation exercises. Training your entire body with exercises like biceps curls, triceps extensions, lateral raises, and calf raises rounds off a training program nicely and balances out your physique development for a better look. However, if a training program uses more machines and isolation exercises than basic compound movements, it won't have anywhere near the impact on caloric expenditure and metabolism.

The exercises you choose also depend a lot on where you train and what equipment you have access to. Where you train is a personal decision. I can't imagine training anywhere but in a well-equipped gym, surrounded by serious lifters and an uplifting atmosphere. You may be different. You might feel uncomfortable working out in a gym, it may not suit your personality, it might be inconvenient for you, or it might not be necessary because you have a home gym.

Regardless of where you train, by all means make use of every piece of equipment you have at your disposal and vary your exercises regularly once you finish the first cycle of this program. You can see some suggestions for variations in the exercise section of this chapter. You might invest in additional equipment for your home gym, or you might consider joining a health club.

The kind of physical condition you're in is another factor that influences

your choice of exercise. There are a number of superbly effective exercises I could teach you, but many of them are advanced movements, requiring a lot of strength or skill to perform and take weeks or months of conditioning to build up to.

Some exercises are superb choices for anyone, but they're very challenging if you're overweight or unconditioned. For example, pull-ups are one of the best exercises you can do for your upper back and upper body pulling muscles. Many beginners and most people who are carrying a lot of excess body weight are unable to perform them. If you can't do pull-ups yet, make it one of your goals and add them to your routine when your weight decreases and your strength increases. A chin-up bar would be a great addition to any home gym.

Warm-up and Joint Mobility

There's a big misconception that stretching and warm-up are the same thing. Static stretching is where you ease into a stretch and hold, to improve your flexibility and increase your range of motion. This type of stretching is not a warm-up and is best performed after your workout, not before. What you should do before your workout is warm up and dynamically loosen up your joints to properly prepare you to transition from the resting state to the exercising state.

The traditional method of warm-up is to hop on a bike or treadmill and ride for five to ten minutes. This raises your body's core temperature, increasing your readiness for exercise. This is known as a general warm-up, and while this method is fine, it's not the best way to prepare for weight training. Using a rowing machine or a full-body elliptical trainer would be a slight improvement because that would involve the upper and lower body.

The ideal approach is to perform joint mobility and dynamic flexibility exercises. These movements not only raise your body temperature like traditional warm-ups, they also wake up the nervous system and prepare the specific joints and muscles you'll be using during the workout. A proper dynamic warm-up also improves your workout performance. A thorough warm-up routine might last six to ten minutes, but this four-minute routine does the job and is perfect for the busy person.

The Body Fat Solution program warm-up, dynamic flexibility, and joint mobility routine: perform all exercises nonstop as a circuit.

1 | Arm circles
15 forward, 15 backward (30 total)

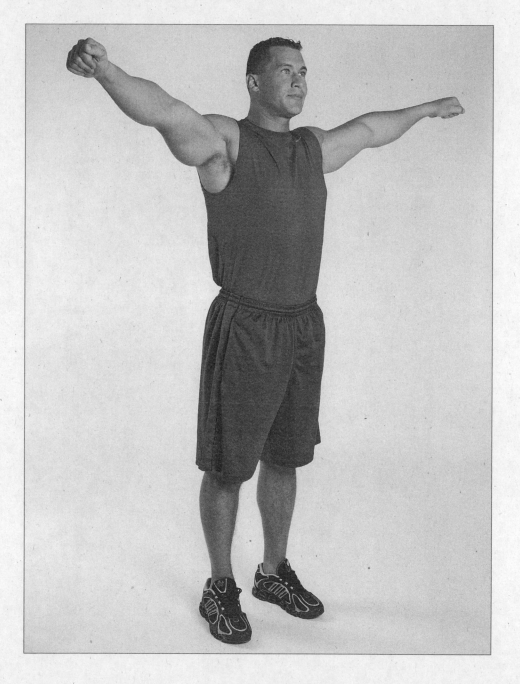

2 | Tai chi twists

15 to each side (30 total)

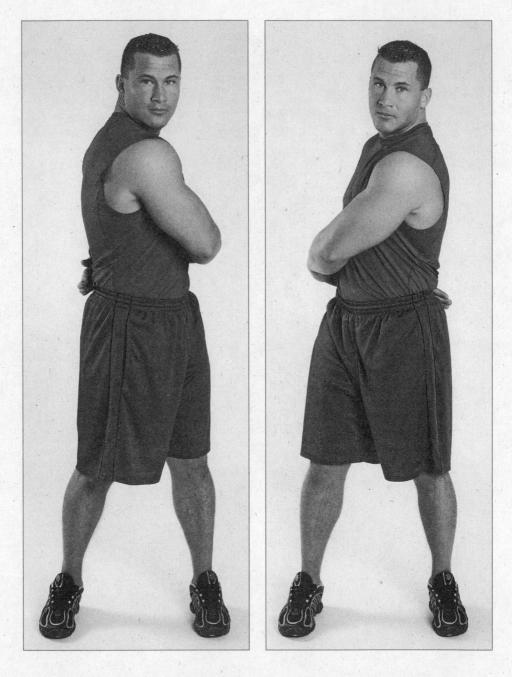

3 | Trunk circles
10 in each direction (20 total)

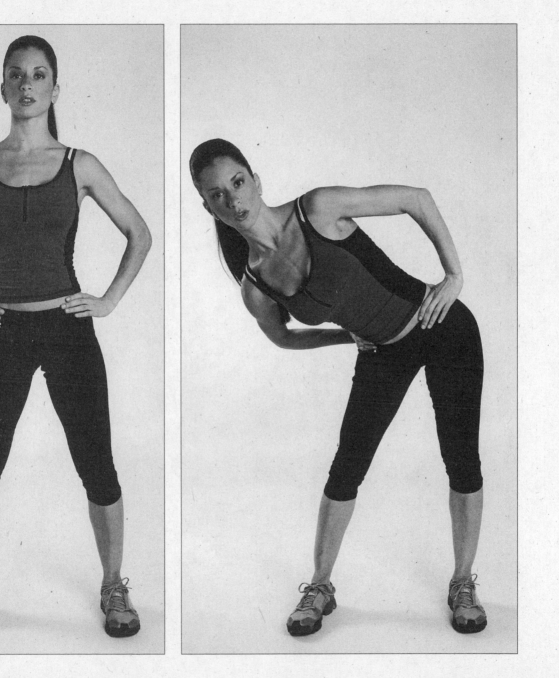

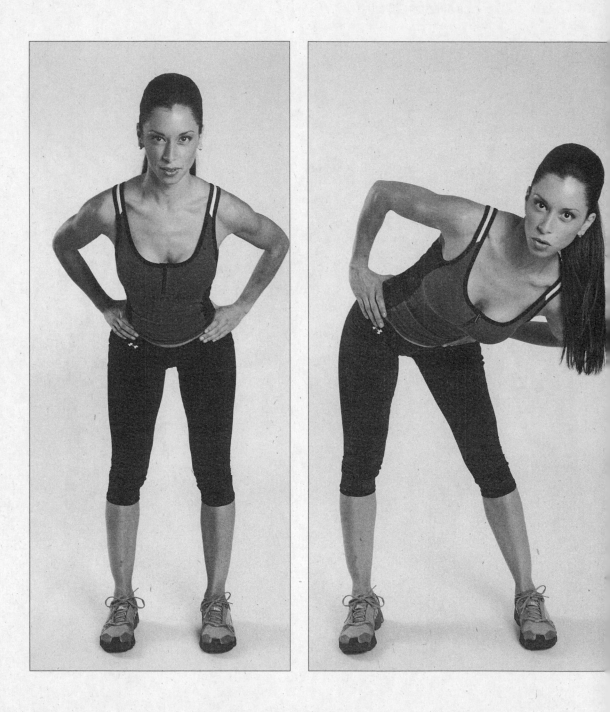

4 | Body-weight prisoner lunges

15 per leg (30 total)

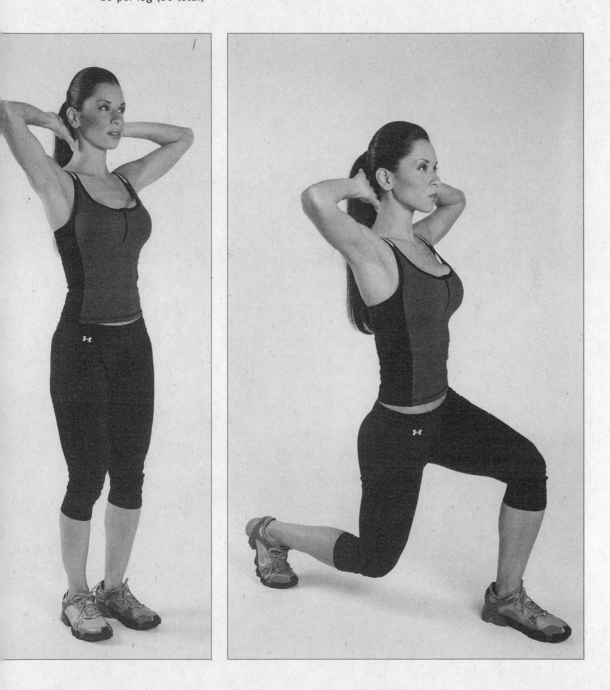

5 | Push-ups or push-ups off knees

15

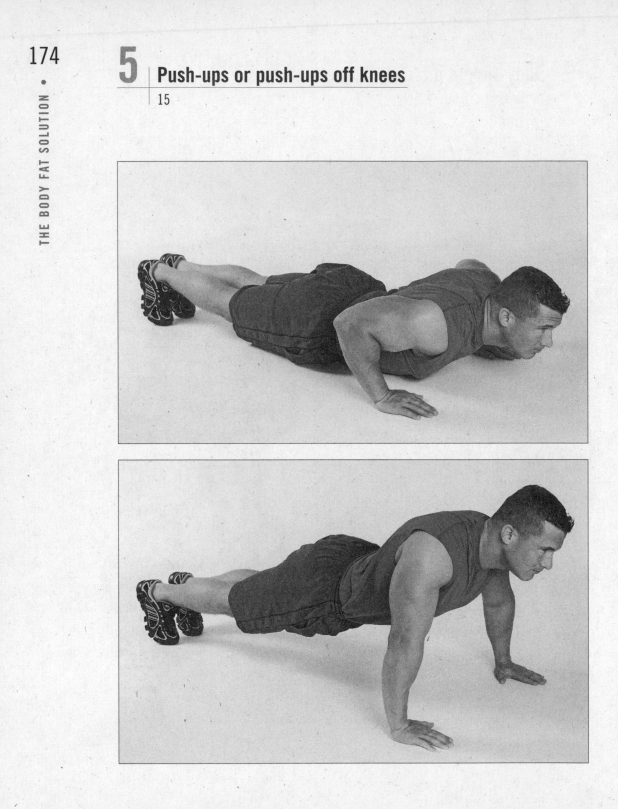

Repetition Maximums and How Much Weight to Lift

Choosing the proper resistance is important, but beginners often have no concept of how much weight to lift or how it's supposed to feel. Once you're comfortable with the exercise technique, then you need to develop a sense for the right amount of weight. One mistake here is simply going through the motions with a weight that's too light to stimulate any muscle growth, strength development, or calorie burning. Although your goal is to progressively lift more weight and get stronger from week to week, it's also foolhardy to try lifting more weight than you can handle in good form.

The easiest way to learn how much weight to lift is to choose a repetition range as a target and then adjust your weight according to that range. With this rep range system, you simply select a weight that allows you to complete at least the minimum number of reps in the range, but no more than the repetition maximum.

For example, during the muscular development and conditioning phase, you choose a weight that you can lift at least twelve times. If you've chosen the right weight, the last two or three reps will be very difficult and you will only be able to do between twelve and fifteen reps. When you can perform fifteen reps or more in good form, that's your cue to increase the weight for your next workout.

Lower reps with more weight increase maximum strength. Medium reps produce maximum muscle development with moderate strength increase. High reps focus more on muscular endurance and metabolic conditioning with little strength. Abdominals and calves may be trained more often in the higher-rep bracket.

Rep category	Rep range	Weight	Benefit
Low	5–7	Heavier	Maximum strength
Medium	8–12	Moderate	Maximum muscle development, some strength
High	13–20	Lighter	Muscular endurance, metabolic conditioning, little strength

Your First Month of Training: The Preconditioning Phase

Your first month of training will be an exciting time when you'll see and feel some amazing changes in your body. When you're a beginner and your body hasn't been subjected to training stress before, you respond to almost anything. It doesn't take a complicated workout program or frequent changes to get results in the beginning.

On the other hand, it's also a time to begin with caution and be mindful not to overdo it. That's why I've set up an introductory four-week workout for first-time beginners. If you have training experience already, you can skip ahead to the second month of training, which is the default training system for the Body Fat Solution program.

The preconditioning phase is designed to gradually expose your body to training stress so you don't get too sore or risk injury. You'll do this by starting with only one set per exercise and then increase to the standard prescription of three sets per exercise by the third week. During the preconditioning period, you will perform all regular straight sets with sixty seconds' rest between each set.

Do adjust the poundage to try to find an ideal ten- to fifteen-rep maximum, but don't worry about breaking any power lifting world records. Instead, focus on perfecting your technique above all else. Breaking bad habits later is a lot more difficult than learning the exercises the right way in the first place.

On Week Four, take your first significant increase in weight to get an idea what it feels like to lift more weight than you are accustomed to. Take your time

Week	Sets	Reps
1	1	10–15
2	2	10–15
3	3	10–15
4	3+ increase resistance	6–10

studying the exercise photographs and reading the exercise descriptions carefully. If in doubt, start on the conservative side in all parameters: sets, reps, intensity of effort, and weight.

A1 Dumbbell squat (or body-weight squats)
B1 Romanian dead lifts
C1 Dumbbell bench press
D1 Dumbbell rows
E1 Reverse crunches

Your Second Month of Training: The Two-Phase System

Your second month is the first "real month" of training in the sense that this will be where the two-phase training program begins. It would take another book to map out a full year of training and illustrate dozens of additional exercises. However, a great feature of the two-phase training system you're learning right here is that it can be used almost indefinitely as a template.

You can continue to use this template as an intermediate trainee with more than three months of training and even as an advanced trainee with a year of experience or more. Unless you change your goals and decide to train for specific purposes such as sports or bodybuilding, then this training schedule won't become outdated. All you have to do is commit yourself to go out there and learn new exercises and new techniques to keep things fresh.

The Body Fat Solution training system is divided into two phases set up in four-week blocks:

PHASE ONE: muscular development and metabolic conditioning
(four weeks/twelve workouts)

Rep range: 12–15   Sets: 3
Rep maximum: 15

PHASE TWO: muscular strength (four weeks/twelve workouts)

Rep range: 6–10   Sets: 3
Rep maximum: 10

Working in distinct phases that focus on different rep ranges is known as periodization. This approach produces better results than programs that give only one repetition prescription, such as three sets of ten, without variation. The reason we've chosen these two rep ranges is because it crosses into all three rep categories. This helps to build strength and develop muscle, while also burning calories and creating favorable metabolic and hormonal adaptations that help increase fat loss.

You will alternate between four-week strength and muscular conditioning phases for all your dumbbell and weight-training exercises. For body-weight exercises such as the bird dog and one-leg hip extensions, you will stay with the higher-rep bracket. Although abdominal exercises can be performed with heavy resistance and periodization, for this program you will also stay with the higher-rep bracket for abdominals. In fact, for abdominals, you can even experiment with reps as high as twenty. When high reps become too easy on body-weight abdominal exercises, it will be time to progress to resisted ab exercises.

Your Weekly Training Schedule

The Body Fat Solution training schedule calls for three workouts per week. You alternate between workout A and workout B. Each workout focuses on the full body but uses different movement patterns. Schedule a full day of rest between each workout, allowing forty-eight hours between sessions and ninety-six hours between training with the same exercises.

Each workout consists of seven to eight exercises, paired in supersets. Extra emphasis is placed on the lower body compound exercises because they produce the greatest increase in energy expenditure and metabolic stimulation. Abs and core exercises are also heavily emphasized because great abs are always one of

Monday	Tuesday	Wednesday	Thursday	Friday	Saturday	Sunday
Workout A	Off	Workout B	Off	Workout A	Off	Off
Workout B	Off	Workout A	Off	Workout B	Off	Off
Workout A	Off	Workout B	Off	Workout A	Off	Off
Workout B	Off	Workout A	Off	Workout B	Off	Off

the most sought-after body parts and a strong core helps protect your lower back from injury.

The most popular weekly schedule is Mondays, Wednesdays, and Fridays with weekends off. If you prefer, you can choose any other three nonconsecutive days per week. Since you're alternating between workouts A and B, the workouts will be staggered every other week. You can perform your cardio training on strength-training days, right after your weights or in a separate session. Or you can do cardio on the days you don't lift, anytime that's convenient for you.

Each phase is four weeks long. After every two phases, you've completed one cycle. At the end of each eight-week cycle, you can change some or all of the exercises and repeat the two-phase cycle again with the new exercises.

The workouts

Most of the exercises in each workout are paired in supersets, identified by A, B, C, and D. You perform the exercises in each superset without resting between them. You do rest, however, for sixty seconds between supersets. A superset pair is indicated by the same letter. For example, A1 and A2 is a superset. Each of the exercises are explained following the workouts. These workouts can be completed in twenty-five to thirty minutes.

Workout A
A1 Dumbbell squat (quads emphasis, lower body)
A2 Bird dog (lower back and glutes)

B1 Dumbbell split squat/static lunge (quads emphasis, lower body)

B2 Dumbbell row (horizontal pull)

C1 Dumbbell bench press (horizontal push)

C2 Plank (core)

D1: One-legged toe raises (calves)

Workout B

A1 Romanian dead lift (hip emphasis, lower body)

A2 Shoulder press (vertical push)

B1 One-legged hip extension (hip dominant, lower body)

B2 Dumbbell pullover (vertical pull)

C1 Reverse crunch (lower abs)

C2 Cross-knee crunch (abs and rotation)

D1 Dumbbell curl (biceps)

D2 Two-dumbbell extension (triceps)

The Two-Cycle Break

Take a week off from weight training every time you complete two eight-week cycles (sixteen weeks). If you're the overachiever type, and you want to continue training, then go ahead, but make it body-weight exercise, calisthenics, light-weight/higher-rep weight training, low-intensity cardio, or some type of recreational exercise. No heavy or high-intensity weight training.

Intermediate Training

The beginner phase lasts for approximately three months; four weeks of preconditioning and then the first eight-week cycle. After you complete the beginner phase, intermediate training lasts from Month Four to Month Twelve. At that point, you'll need to begin changing your exercises and progress to more difficult exercises and other methods that progressively challenge you.

Advanced Training and Beyond

There are no secret or magical workout programs, only training principles that follow unbreakable laws of physics and human physiology. If you understand the basic principles of overload and adaptation, then you will understand that almost any training program will work for a while, but no program works for long. Eventually your body will adapt to everything. In that sense, variety is the spice of your training life.

After you hit the advanced level with a year of training under your belt, one thing that will change is how often you vary your program. As an advanced trainee, your body adapts more quickly, so you should change your exercises every four weeks, instead of every eight weeks.

You should also begin learning new combinations of exercises and other lifting techniques. If you don't know any other exercises or advanced techniques, then go forth and learn some. Not sure where to start? A great resource is the Body Fat Solution website at www.TheBodyFatSolution.com. Don't consider this Body Fat Solution training program as the be-all and end-all. This is really only the beginning of a lifelong learning experience and adventure in self-improvement.

The Exercises

Each exercise has a specific purpose and develops particular muscular functions. Each exercise entry consists of photographs showing the proper form and includes a written description of how you should perform the exercise. Be sure to read the entire description because there are points of exercise technique you'll miss if you only look at the pictures. Every repetition should be performed in a controlled fashion, especially the "eccentric" portion of the movement, where you lower the weight and the muscle lengthens.

The dumbbell squat

Place your feet slightly wider than shoulder-width apart, toes pointing forward or angled slightly outward. Holding dumbbells in each hand on the outside of each leg, begin the movement by breaking at the hips and squat down as if you were going to sit in a chair. Drop to parallel or slightly below parallel, keeping your head up and your back flat or slightly arched (do not round over your back). Using the quadricep and hip muscles, stand back up to the start position.

■ **Alternates:** dumbbell front squat, dumbbell sumo squat, static lunge, step-up, one-legged squat.

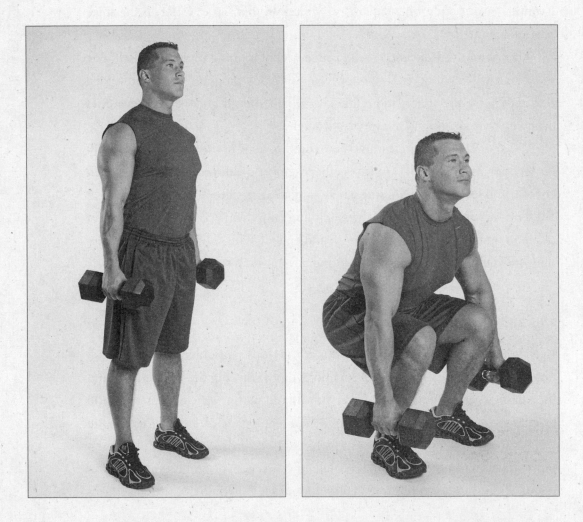

Bird dog

Kneel on a mat or soft surface on your hands and knees. Simultaneously raise your right arm and left leg, keeping your abdominals braced. At the top of the movement, your right arm and left leg should be fully extended to form a straight line from hand to foot. Hold momentarily at the top position and repeat on the other side. Performed properly, this exercise is more challenging than it may look.

■ **Alternates:** cobras, reverse hyperextensions, hyperextensions.

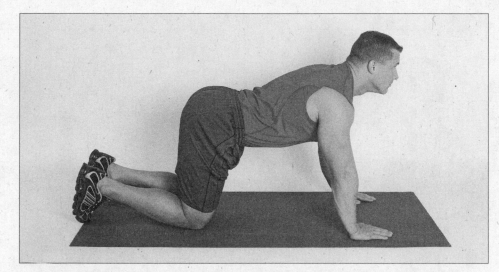

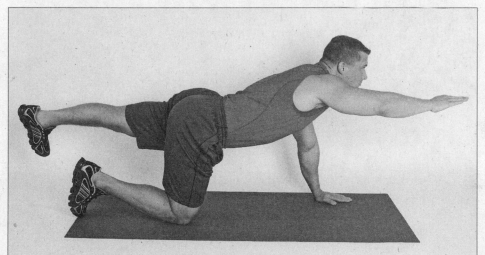

The dumbbell split squat (static lunge)

Holding a dumbbell in each hand on the outside of your legs, step forward with your right leg into the lunge position. Adjust your left foot behind you if necessary until you feel balanced. Slowly squat down on your right leg, focusing on the left knee dropping straight down to the floor. Push back up to the start position, but do not stand all the way up. Keep your right knee bent the entire time. As you perform each rep, keep your head up, chest up, and torso as vertical as possible (do not lean forward).

■ **Alternates:** dumbbell front squat, dumbbell sumo squat, Bulgarian split squat, step-up.

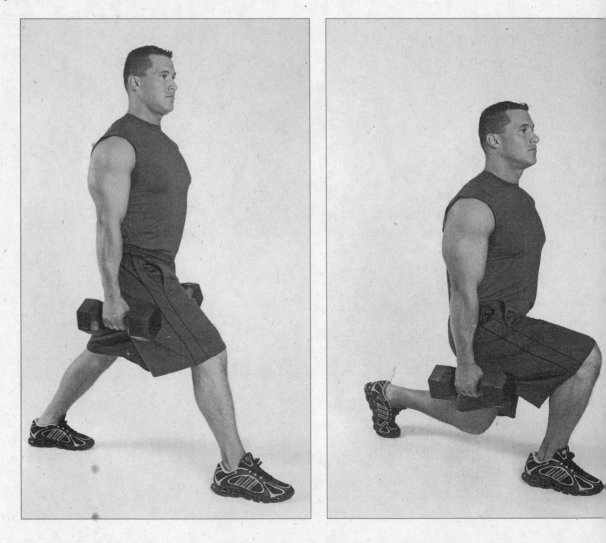

Dumbbell Romanian dead lift

Stand with your feet shoulder-width apart, toes pointing forward. Hold two dumbbells in front of your thighs, palms facing toward your legs. Keep your knees unlocked and slightly bent throughout the movement. Bend forward at the waist, keeping your head up and your butt out. Maintain a flat back as you lower the weights. Lower the dumbbells to about mid-shin height, or as your hamstring flexibility allows. Stop the movement if your back rounds. Skip this exercise if you have any spinal or lower back injury and stop immediately if you feel any lower back pain.

■ **Alternates:** barbell Romanian dead lift, one-legged Romanian dead lift, Swiss ball leg curl, dumbbell between feet leg curl, lying leg curl machine, seated leg curl machine.

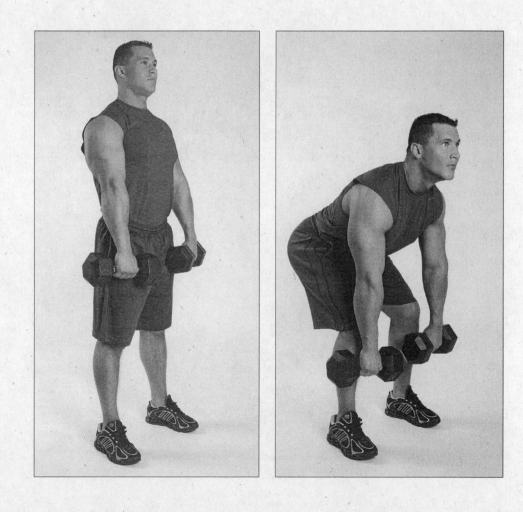

One-legged hip extension

Lie on your back with your knees bent and your feet flat on the floor. Straighten out your left leg completely, while keeping your right leg planted firmly on the floor. Using your glute muscles, lift your hips up off the floor until your body forms a straight line, keeping your abs braced. Lower your hips back down slowly, but not all the way to the floor.

■ **Alternates:** two-legged hip extension, glute-ham raise, hyperextension, reverse hyperextension.

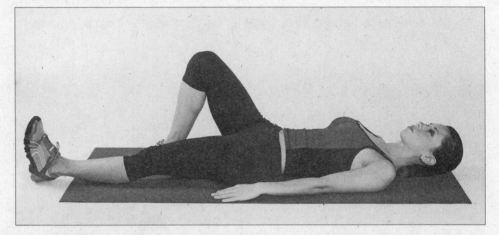

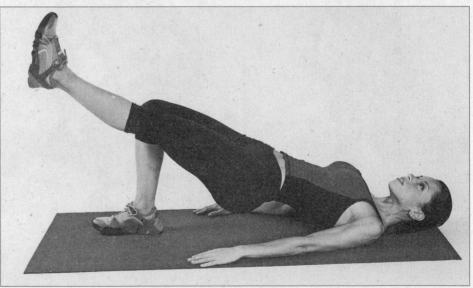

Plank

Lie on your stomach on an exercise mat or carpeted surface. Prop your body up on your forearms and position your body in a straight line from head to feet. Hold the straight line position with your body several inches off the floor for 30–60 seconds.

■ **Alternates:** side plank, plank off a Swiss ball, one-legged plank.

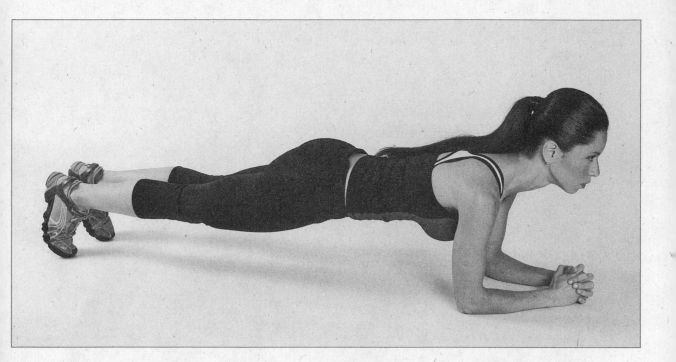

One-legged calf raise

Stand on the edge of a step, a block of wood, or a thick book with the ball of your right foot on the edge. Holding a dumbbell in your right hand, rise up on the ball of your foot as high as you can go. Drop your heel below the edge until you feel a slight stretch in your calf. If you don't have a step or block of wood or book to stand on, simply perform the exercise off the floor, as pictured. Repeat for the desired number of reps, then without stopping; switch to the left leg and repeat.

■ **Alternates:** standing calf machine, seated calf machine.

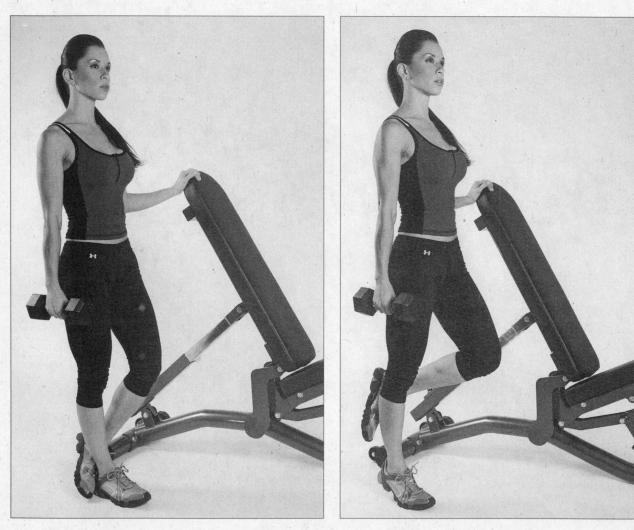

Dumbbell bench press

Grab a set of dumbbells and lie on your back on a bench. Begin with the dumbbells at arm's length over your chest, palms facing toward your feet. Lower the dumbbells to the sides of your chest, then press them back up to the starting position.

■ **Alternates:** push-ups, barbell bench press, incline bench press.

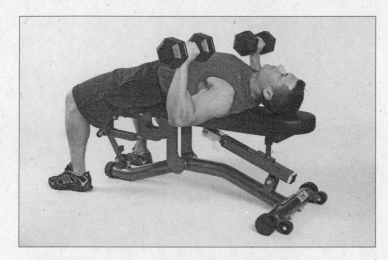

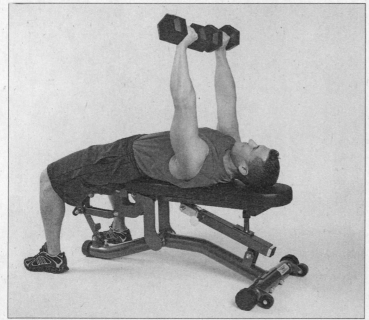

Dumbbell shoulder press

Grab a set of dumbbells and sit on the edge of a bench or chair. Begin with the dumbbells at shoulder height with your palms facing away from your body. Press the dumbbells up until your arms are straight overhead. Slowly lower back to the starting position. This exercise can also be done standing.

■ **Alternate:** barbell shoulder press.

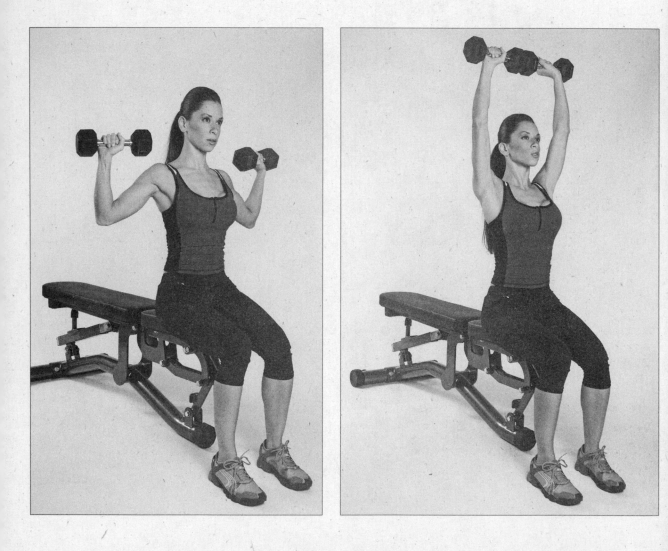

Dumbbell rows

Grab a dumbbell with your right hand and place your left hand and left knee on a bench. From arm length, bend your elbow and pull the dumbbell up toward your waist. Keep your palm facing your body. Keeping your head up and back flat throughout the exercise, slowly lower the dumbbell back down until your arm is straight and you feel a stretch.

■ **Alternates:** seated cable row, barbell row, inverted row.

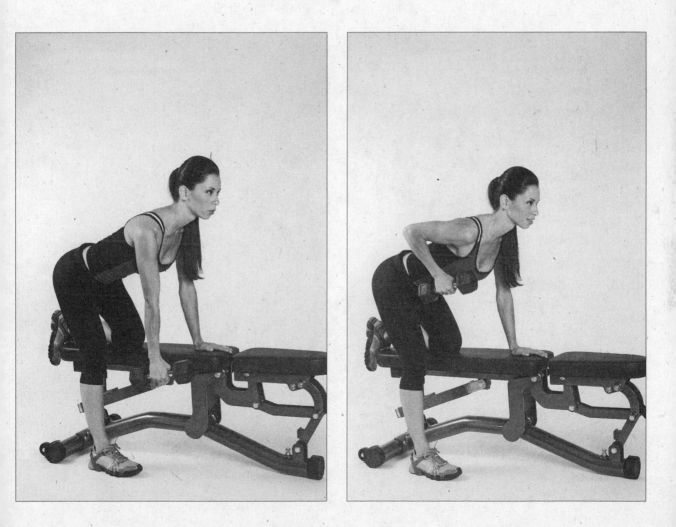

Two-dumbbell pullover

Grab two dumbbells and lie flat on your back on a bench. Very slowly lower the dumbbells behind your head, until you begin to feel a slight stretch in the lat muscles under your armpits. Pull the dumbbells at arm's length over your face and back to the starting position over your chest. Keep your elbows slightly bent, but maintain that locked arm position throughout the movement.

■ **Alternates:** single dumbbell pullover, pull-ups, pulldowns, pullover machine.

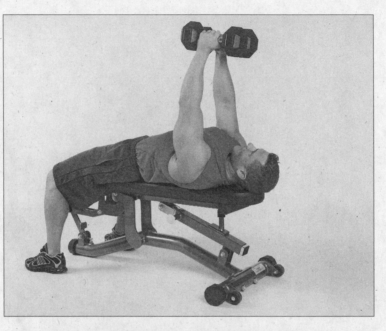

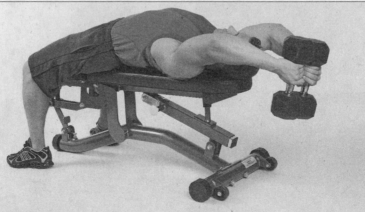

Reverse crunch

Lie flat on your back on a mat or soft surface with your feet in the air, knees bent at a 90-degree angle, and hips bent at a 90-degree angle. Place your hands underneath your hips or flat on the floor to your sides. Gently, using the abdominal muscles, rock your knees back over your chest or far enough so your hips roll up off the floor. Return slowly to start position with control, using the abdominal muscles.

■ **Alternates:** hip lifts, incline reverse crunches, hanging knee-up, hanging leg raises.

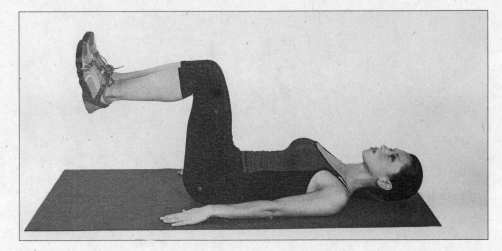

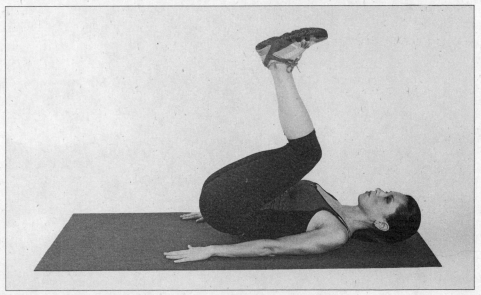

Cross-knee crunch

Lie flat on your back on a mat or soft surface with your knees bent and feet flat on the floor. Place your left foot across your right knee. Crunch across your body, right elbow to left knee. After completing prescribed number of reps on the right side, switch sides and repeat.

■ **Alternates:** Swiss ball crunch, cable woodchopper, dumbbell woodchopper, upper-body Russian twists, lower-body Russian twists.

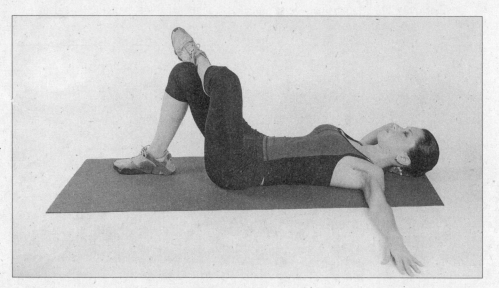

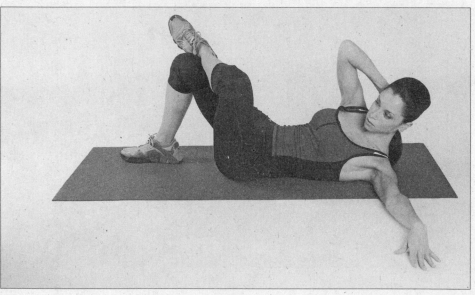

Dumbbell curls

Take a shoulder-width stance, holding a dumbbell in each hand with your palms facing up. Curl both dumbbells up together to shoulder height. At the top of the movement, your palms should be facing your body. Hold the contraction briefly and squeeze the biceps, then slowly return the dumbbells to the starting position. Keep your torso vertical and avoid leaning backward.

■ **Alternates:** barbell curls, incline dumbbell curls, preacher bench curls.

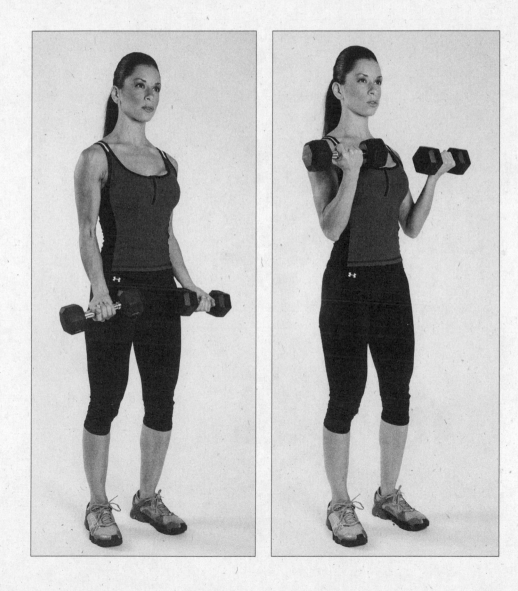

Two-dumbbell triceps extensions

Lie on your back on a bench holding two dumbbells at arm's length over your upper chest or face. Bend at the elbows and slowly lower both dumbbells together along the sides of your forehead. When your arms are bent at a 90-degree angle, extend your arms back up to the starting position.

- **Alternates:** dumbbell extension behind the head, dumbbell kickbacks, triceps cable pushdowns, close grip bench press, parallel bar dips.

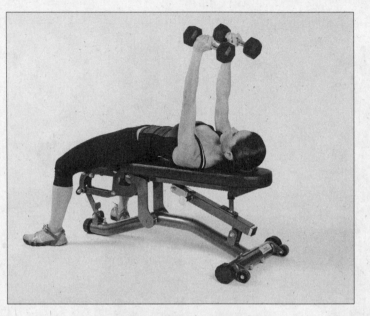

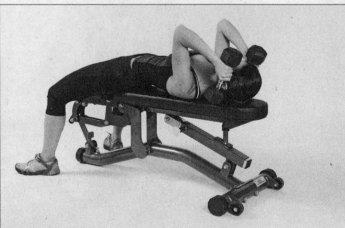

The Social Support Solution

Recruiting Friends, **Family**, Peers, and **Mentors** into Your **Support** Circle

> WE are all being influenced by someone. Since this influence will determine, to some extent, the direction of our lives, it is far better to deliberately choose the people we will permit to influence us than to allow the power of the wrong influence to weave its effect on us without our knowledge or conscious choice.
>
> —JIM ROHN, MOTIVATIONAL SPEAKER AND AUTHOR

So far you've learned: You are what you think. You are what you believe. You are what you eat. You are the exercise you get. Now, let's add another: You are the company you keep.

If it hasn't happened already, you're slowly but surely becoming just like the people you spend the most time with. Motivational writer Charlie "Tremendous" Jones says that you will be the same person in five years except for two things: the people you meet and the books you read.

197

We usually don't realize how much we're being influenced by our friends, family, and coworkers because the influence is subtle and the effects are gradual. Yet it's those little nudges and small temptations that can do the most damage, because they add up over time and you don't notice them or appreciate their impact.

A friend says, "Have another beer." Your coworker leaves doughnuts on your desk every morning. You take clients out for drinks and dinner several times per week. Your mom says, "Have seconds, I made it just for you!" Your training partner doesn't show up, so you skip the workout as well. Your spouse criticizes your new fitness goals. Your college buddies keep you out late partying. Little by little, it all adds up. Then one day you wake up and say, "What happened? How did my health slip so far? How did I gain all this weight?"

There's an old parable about the little bird and the crow. The little bird was covering one eye and crying hysterically. An owl landed nearby and said, "What's wrong, little bird?"

The little bird moved its wing, exposing a gaping wound where it once had an eye.

"I see," hooted the owl, "you're crying because the mean old crow pecked out your eye!"

"No," the bird replied bitterly, "I'm not crying because the crow pecked out my eye, I'm crying because I let him peck out my eye."

The people in your social circle and how you let them affect you will have a greater influence on the direction of your life than any other factor. Nowhere do personal associations influence you more than in your quest for optimal health and a better body. In fact, social influence is so powerful, it can even override biological hunger.

Most people eat more when in groups, especially if tasty food is readily available, as in restaurants, buffets, picnics, or holiday dinners. Usually, the larger the group, the more you'll eat and the more likely you'll be to drink. If everyone at the table is eating dessert, you're more likely to eat dessert too, even if you're already stuffed. Psychologists call it "social facilitation."

Eating with others, however, can also restrain food intake, depending on who your companions are. If you think others are observing and evaluating you, you'll make better choices and eat less food. This is called "impression management." Whether your dining companion is your trainer, an accountability partner, or even a first date, if they're watching you and you care what they think, you're on your best behavior.

The Social Influence Inventory: Who's Influencing You?

Most people have no idea how much of their behavior has developed as a result of modeling the people they spend time with. As human beings, we have an automatic tendency to conform to the words, behaviors, and habits of the people who surround us. When you become aware of which people in your life are positive influences and which are negative, that's the beginning of a life transformation.

You start by taking an inventory of all the people in your life. Who do you spend the most time with? What kind of influence are they having on you? Is that influence helping you move toward your goals or away from them? Based on your answers, you'll be able to place all the people in your life into one of two categories and decide who to spend more time with and who to spend less time with.

THE TURKEYS AND THE CROWS

The pessimist. Pessimists find the negative side of everything. They see the glass half empty, they always expect the worst, and they never expect to succeed. These turkeys are everywhere, and while they're usually not malicious, be wary. Negative attitudes are contagious and prolonged exposure can be hazardous.

The complainer. Complainers are always whining about something. They go out of their way to tell everyone within earshot everything that's wrong with their bodies, their health, their lives, other people, and the world. Complainers usually aren't dangerous, but they are draining. They'll wear you down emotionally if you stay around them for long.

The critic. The critic is an expert at what you're doing wrong, even though he may have no experience giving him the right to speak into your life. He'll tell you what's wrong with your diet, what's wrong with your training, and if you're doing great, he'll say it would have been better if you'd done it another way. Beware also of the well-meaning critic. Her criticism appears constructive, but often comes from jealousy or envy when she sees you pulling away from the pack: "Haven't you lost enough weight already? Don't you know that being too lean is unhealthy?"

The hedonist. The hedonist is that jolly, fun-loving guy whose motto is "Life is too short, live a little!" Ironically, his life often *is* short because of the lifestyle he's chosen. Be careful of the hedonist, who seems the most harmless of the bunch since he's such a happy character. But he's also the person most likely to recruit you to join him in living fast and dying young because he doesn't pressure you, he entices you with fun.

The temptress. "Mmmm, this chocolate is to die for." "Loosen up, have a glass of wine with me." "These cookies are sinful, you have to try one." These are the siren songs of the temptress. She's always dangling an indulgent lure and egging you on to take it. She baits you to partake of scrumptious snacks, decadent desserts, or alcoholic drinks. If you don't join her, she eats in front of you. Even if you're the strong type, be on guard because the temptress persuades with gastronomic seduction.

The dream destroyer. Dream destroyers are the ones who hear your plans and immediately shoot them down. Not only will they say your plans are dumb, they'll tell you they're impossible and can't be done at all. These people are dangerous. If it weren't for the visionaries who carry on in spite of dream destroyers, innovation would cease, exploration would end, and human progress would grind to a halt.

The saboteur. Saboteurs are the worst kind of people to allow in your life because they attack, ridicule, belittle, and undermine your efforts. A pessimist or complainer may be a good-hearted person, even a friend, who has simply developed a negative attitude. Saboteurs are deliberately malicious. They aim to knock you down and get satisfaction in seeing you fall.

THE EAGLES AND THE OWLS

The optimist. The optimists see the bright side of everything. To them, there's a hidden benefit in every adversity, a lesson in every failure, a silver lining in every dark cloud. Those are the optimist's credos. Optimists radiate positive energy. It's uplifting to be around them.

The complimenter. The complimenter looks for the good in you and goes out of her way to tell you about it. She notices little details, from your hair to your shoes. If you lost a few ounces, she'd notice. Few things feel as good as being with a complimenter. Few people are more important in your life when you're struggling with physical change.

The cheerleader. Cheerleaders pump you up, encourage you, motivate you, and celebrate your successes with you. "You can do it" is their motto. Although they might not go out of their way to give tangible support, they're usually attentive listeners and pillars of emotional support.

The accountability partner. This is who you answer to. If you take a wrong turn that leads into temptation, he'll nudge you back on the straight and narrow. He won't take excuses, he'll only accept results. If you say you're going to do it, your partner will hold you to it.

The coach. Coaches are trainers, teachers, and mentors, but also much more. The coach is a liberator of human potential. He helps you see your potential and helps bring out the best in you. He's not afraid to push you. His feedback is honest. His criticism is constructive. When you're doing well, he's quick to praise you. When you veer off course, he's quick to correct you.

The emotional supporter. This is the friend who's always there to comfort you. If you're feeling down, she'll lift your spirits. In moments of weakness, she'll give you strength. In times of doubt, she'll bolster your confidence. When there's no one else to talk to, she'll lend you her ears and you'll always feel safe in telling her how you feel.

The dreamers. "The dreamers are the saviors of the world," said James Allen, the inspirational writer. These are the builders, the creators and the biggest of thinkers. To the dreamer, anything is possible. Their goals are so big, their ambitions so high, that even the optimists sometimes raise an eyebrow. If you have a dreamer in your life, you are the luckiest person alive.

Four Strategies to Deal with Negative Relationships

How does your support circle stack up? If you're surrounded by eagles, then congratulations. Cherish those relationships. Nurture them. They are your lifeline. If you're surrounded by turkeys, don't feel bad. Most people are. No matter what your social influence inventory revealed, there are ways to handle every situation. Here are the four best strategies to deal with the negatives.

1. Limit your exposure to the negatives

The directive is simple: spend less time with pessimists, critics, and other negative people. You can't completely avoid or quickly remove some people, such as complaining, energy-draining coworkers, from your life, but you can reduce your exposure to them.

A good first step is to begin placing an extraordinarily high value on your time. As you start to realize that time is life itself and you have a limited supply, you'll begin to have less tolerance for time wasters. It will start becoming very easy not to voluntarily subject yourself to their presence any longer than necessary.

In the office, there are three important words you need to memorize: "back to work." Whenever someone negative intrudes on your work space, tell him you have to get back to work. It's the perfect exit strategy. By socializing less and work-ing more, you'll also get more work done. Who knows, you might get promoted right out of the turkey pen into your own private office.

2. Increase your exposure to the positives

At the same time that you decrease your exposure to negative people, you can increase your exposure to positive people. Rearrange your time and priorities to expand the positive associations in your life. Do anything it takes to share time with winners and strengthen your relationships with them. If you can be person-ally mentored by an eagle, go out of your way to do it. Get up early, spend money, travel, intern, volunteer—anything.

A spoonful of positive energy can counteract a truckload of negative energy. One sincere compliment from a friend can keep your attitude up and your eating on track all day long. A phone call with a coach could keep you account-able for an entire week as you anticipate your next weigh-in. One inspiring mo-ment with a dreamer could leave an impact on you that lasts a lifetime.

3. Build immunity from the negatives

Expecting to eliminate all negativity from your life is unrealistic. If you're going to spend time out in the world, you must develop immunity from criticism and shield yourself from negative energy. If you took every criticism to heart or gave up every time someone told you to quit, you wouldn't get to first base.

Many years ago, I learned a simple daily ritual from Tom Hopkins, an inter-nationally renowned sales trainer and motivational speaker. Tom said that to be successful, especially in a field like sales where you face rejection and criticism daily, you can never let other people steal your energy. You must also avoid gos-sip, jealousy, anger, and negative thinking.

To keep these negative forces from getting under your skin, every morning before you go to work or out into the world, you put yourself inside a force field of positive energy. Visualize yourself stepping into it and saying, "Zip, zip. I am now in my positive shell." If negative energy starts flying your way, you can watch it bounce right off you and back where it came from.

4. Avoid the negatives completely

Staying in the presence of toxic people who ridicule you and undermine your efforts is like committing slow suicide. It's better to be alone than in the company of dream destroyers and saboteurs. One decision is always clear: malicious people must be pruned from your life like weeds from a garden.

Other relationships can be more difficult to sever. Prime example: your drinking buddies. You may have known them for years and shared many laughs and good times. They've always been well-meaning and they've never been malicious. But the influence of some friends can become negative just the same. An occasional drink may do little harm, but alcohol and late nights never got anyone healthier, leaner, or more successful.

What to do? Tell your friends about your goals. Tell them you'd love it if they'd join you in the gym. You'll still join them for company. But you won't join them in the bars. Do they ridicule your new lifestyle choices or pressure you to keep drinking? If so, then this decision also becomes clear. To fulfill your potential, you have to avoid negative influences, sometimes even your old friends.

Five Types of Support You Need

What exactly does support mean? This isn't a question to take lightly, because if you don't know what support is, and what support means to you, you won't know if you're receiving it and you won't be able to express your needs to others.

There are five types of social support.

1. Emotional Support

Emotional support is a pair of sympathetic and empathetic ears. Emotional support is a shoulder to lean on or cry on. Emotional support is when you know another person hears you, is concerned for you, and cares about you. The benefits are not just psychological. Emotional support has a proven stress-buffering effect. Scientific evidence published in *The Journal of Biological Psychiatry* has demonstrated that emotional social support reduces the physical effects of stress and lowers levels of the stress hormone, cortisol.

2. Educational Support

We are more emotional than logical creatures, but emotional support isn't enough. Without an education in exercise physiology and nutrition, you'd have no way to create effective nutrition and training strategies. You'd continue to believe in myths, fall for the latest baloney, and jump on the newest diet bandwagons. Fortunately, educational support is the easiest type to find because you can get it from books and directly from mentors and coaches. The tricky part is knowing what to read and who to listen to. (Hint: You're doing pretty good right now.)

3. Appraisal Support

Social psychologists have discovered that regardless of where support comes from, the "how am I doing" type of support is the kind most likely to help you take weight off and keep it off. This is known as appraisal support. Honest appraisal isn't always easy to get because those who care about you don't want to hurt your feelings. Sometimes the truth hurts, but you need to hear it, anyway. And it might need to come from a drill-sergeant, taskmaster of a coach. Someone needs to tell you, "You're not doing so good. Get your butt moving!" Once in motion, then you need someone to tell you, "Good job, you're heading the right way," or "You're off course, let's adjust your direction."

4. Tangible Support

Sometimes words or empathy aren't enough. Sometimes you need physical support that only comes through another person's actions. For example, a supportive partner might go food shopping with you or for you. They give you a ride to the gym, train with you, or tag along to spot you and motivate you. They might babysit your kids while you're working out. Or they provide any other type of tangible support that's more than words. Tangible support can also come in the form of a personal trainer kicking your butt in the gym.

5. Accountability Support

Accountability is when people check up on each other to make sure they've taken the actions they promised to take, fulfilled the commitments they made, and met the goals they set. I'm convinced that external accountability is one of the most powerful forms of support as well as motivation. Whom are you accountable to? Whom do you report to? Whom do you answer to? Ask these questions often. If the answer is "no one," then ask, "Whom *can* I be accountable to, and how soon can I start?"

Getting Support from Your Natural Social Network

To fully leverage the power of social support, you're going to need all five types of support at one time or another. But where do you get it? The logical place to start is right where you are now, with the people already in your life, also known as your natural network. If necessary, you can get support from outside your natural network, but start where you are now, with your closest friends and family. If they're negative, pessimistic, or simply aren't giving you the support you need yet, don't call them turkeys or walk out on them. Ask for support and give them a chance to help.

Family

Family support can be tricky because food and family are so closely linked. "You've hardly touched your plate." "Have seconds." "Aren't you having dessert?" "What's the matter, you don't like my cooking?" Who hasn't felt this kind of pressure at the dinner table, and geez, how do you say no to your mom? (Actually, it's simple, just put the letters *n* and *o* together—trust me, she'll still love you.)

Although your family can act like turkeys at times, the good news is formal research and personal surveys both consistently reveal that your family is likely to be your best source of support if you appeal to them for help. One study from the University of Michigan reported that 73 percent of subjects said their families or spouses were their most helpful resource in their efforts to lose weight, while only 15 percent said their friends were most helpful.

If your family is unsupportive, then reach out for help from other sources like friends, neighbors, coworkers, and fitness professionals, but keep faith in your family. They may come around when they see you start to change. As you become a leader, role model, and source of positive energy, you may be surprised at how *you* begin to influence *them*.

Spouse or Significant Other

When Scott turned up the intensity level in his weight lifting program, along with starting a highly structured new meal plan, Angie, his wife of seven years, started making comments like these: "Why do you always have to go to extremes with these fitness goals? Is it really necessary to eat such expensive health foods? Did you really have to buy another training book?" Scott not only felt unsupported, he felt like he was being sabotaged. Oddly enough, he never asked her to join him. He thought she already had a nice figure. Since she wasn't complaining about how she looked, he wasn't paying attention to her cries for help and her desire to start training again the way she did before the kids arrived.

As Scott was heading out to the gym, Angie would say things like, "It must be nice to get out of the house." Again, he felt attacked, but what she was really saying was, "I'd like to join you." One day, Angie mentioned that her job wasn't challenging and she needed a goal and some other way to feel more satisfaction and accomplishment. Finally, the lightbulb went on and Scott got the message. "I wasn't listening to her or asking her the right questions," he realized. "I now see that it wasn't the leaner, sexier body she wanted the most. That was just a bonus. What she really wanted was the mental and emotional boost she got from pursuing and achieving fitness goals. She wanted to feel successful, proud, empowered, and disciplined."

To support each other fully, you must communicate clearly. This means listening, asking, and speaking each other's language. Ask your significant other if he or she wants to join you on your fitness journey. Share your goals and your emotional reasons why. If necessary, help each other set goals and be sure to include outcome goals like ideal body weight as well as daily action goals. Hold each other accountable for daily actions and weekly results. Measure progress and ask "How am I doing?" often.

Children

In a pilot study from the University of Michigan on social networks and social support in weight loss, 71 percent of the participants said their children were a negative influence on their own weight control. That's why, if you have kids, involving them in your health and fitness program is important to your own success. It's also important to their futures.

Childhood obesity has become as serious an epidemic as adult obesity. Children who develop poor health habits at a young age are far more predisposed to become overweight as adults. Peer influence doesn't affect only whether someone drinks alcohol or takes drugs. A new study from the University of Miami published in the *The Journal of Pediatric Research* says that affiliation with a reference group (such as "jocks," "populars," "burnouts," and "brains") is directly related to an adolescent's eating, exercise, and weight control behaviors.

Peer influence affects all of us at every age, but adolescence is a crucial time when we can help young people understand the importance of their reference group and give them good role models. You may already know this, but in light of the confirming research, your children give you one more motivation, one more reason why you should diligently live the fitness lifestyle. Even though peers are a major influence on adolescents, the number one authority figure and role model in a young person's life is his or her parents.

Siblings

Some of the strongest accountability and training partnerships I have ever seen were among siblings. James and Terri, who are members of my online Burn the Fat Inner Circle group, are a brother-and-sister team who lost seventy-three and twenty-five pounds of fat, respectively, by teaming up to support each other.

About their partnership, James said, "I do have a competitive personality and there was some friendly sibling rivalry. If Terri had better results than I did on any given week, that would push me to do a little better the next week. I think being accountable to my sister was easier than being accountable to anyone else. I was more comfortable discussing the details of my poor physical condition with a family member, and since she was on the same program, she knew exactly what I was going through."

Terri agreed that their collaboration was instrumental in keeping each other away from temptation. "There were a couple of times when I fell into old habits and had an extra cheat meal midweek. When weighing and body fat measuring day came around, my weekly numbers weren't as good as they should have been, so I had to confess. James reminded me that it wasn't worth sacrificing an entire week of hard work for a badly timed cheat meal. By being honest with James we were both able to learn from those experiences."

Friends

Like family, friends can be your most helpful source of support. But depending on who you hang out with, they may also be the greatest source of pressure to indulge in unhealthy habits. Out of every type of relationship, mutual friends have the strongest influence on each other's behaviors and lifestyles. That's why it's so important to cultivate and strengthen all your supportive friendships.

The great thing about friends is that they can be your key source of emotional support. That's important because you can't get that kind of support anywhere. Of course, you may have different types of friends and it's ideal to enlist the support of more than one. Certain friends may be especially empathetic, while others you may depend on for advice. Also, if you lean on one person too much, it can be draining to them and if they're unavailable, you may feel unsupported. Share your goals with all your friends and ask them to hold you accountable. When you achieve them, celebrate together.

When you start becoming successful, you may find that you naturally gravitate away from certain friends, because you no longer resonate with each other. Others may accuse you of "forgetting where you came from" or being "too good for them" because they feel left behind. If you feel guilty about that and you're tempted to fall back into their lower energy, you need to do a reframe: you haven't left anyone behind; some of your friends chose to stay behind and accept mediocrity. You'd gladly welcome them back in your life if they would climb up and stand beside you. See who stands by you through challenges and changes and then you'll know who your true friends are.

Neighbors

Although friends and neighbors are often one and the same, many people don't think about reaching out to neighbors for help. When you do, you may find your most supportive partners in success are right next door. In numerous social support studies, neighbors were rated as more supportive than family. Maybe they won't become the "cry on their shoulder" type of emotional support partners, but they sure make great walking, hiking, jogging, or cycling partners. Just walk out your front door, knock on theirs, and the two of you are off and running.

Coworkers

Your workplace often creates an interesting dilemma. Some of your coworkers may be the worst saboteurs and energy vampires in your life. Others may be your greatest allies. The problem is, unless you change your job, you have to deal with both of them. This is one of those situations where you must use the immunity and limited exposure strategies to reduce their impact on you, while simultaneously expanding your association with positive coworkers.

Support *is* available at work. Take advantage of it. You can make new friends, find training partners, and utilize fitness facilities. Fitness competitions at work are more popular than ever and many companies are offering corporate health and fitness programs, including paid gym memberships and incentives. They know that healthy employees are better performers who take fewer sick days, which lowers their health care costs.

My friend Ryan says he's been more consistent with his workouts than ever since he started using the gym at work. He said it had all the equipment and amenities as his old public gym, but was far more convenient. One of the benefits: he got in the best shape of his life for his wedding and honeymoon in Mexico. (Of course, the nutrition coaching he got from me helped too.)

Recruiting Support by Expanding Your Social Network

Not getting the support you need from your existing social network? No worries. Support doesn't end there. Reach out and expand your social network to provide any support that's missing.

You may need to expand your network for educational support. Your friends and family might be your best source of emotional support but your worst source of how-to advice. If information is the type of help you need, don't hesitate to get professional help in the form of a trainer, coach, commercial support group, or online community.

Hire a Trainer

Many people prefer to exercise alone. They train with their own style, in their private space, at their own pace. However, having a trainer offers tremendous advantages. Personal trainers offer accountability, appraisal, education, and tangible support. In terms of physical results, a professionally designed workout program can beat the pants off a poorly designed program, while keeping you free from injury. Regular changes in the program also help prevent you from getting bored or falling into old habit patterns.

A trainer also provides the highest degree of accountability. Things get done when discipline is imposed externally and high expectations are set. There's also an extra motivational factor involved that makes every person want to push harder when someone is watching. When that someone is a coach or trainer, I call it "the drill sergeant effect." This effect is even more powerful if there are real consequences—emotional, financial, or physical—for falling short on goals and not fulfilling expectations.

Enroll in a Group Fitness Class

Speaking of military metaphors, is it any coincidence that "boot camp" classes and group personal training are more popular than ever before? Take a group class where you're not one-on-one with a trainer but with a group. Not only is your "drill sergeant" or "tough love" instructor watching you, your group peers are also watching you. What happens if you stop short or quit in front of everyone? Does the prospect of pushing yourself harder seem more likely?

Find a Training Partner

In the mid-1970s, Arnold Schwarzenegger was the most successful bodybuilder in the world, having won Mr. Olympia six times. Arnold credited his success to one thing more than any other. "The biggest help I ever had was a training partner," he said. "I wrote more stories about training partners in the magazines than anything else because I felt that this was one of the most important subjects to talk about. If you don't have a training partner, you actually get only fifty percent out of your physique."

Arnold explained that we all have physical and emotional ups and downs.

No matter how disciplined and dedicated we are, there are going to be down days when our attitude is negative and we find all kinds of excuses. It's on those days that your training partner has the responsibility to lift you up to his state. If you don't have a training partner, you might skip the workout altogether, or do your workout halfheartedly.

Your choice of a training partner is paramount. Choose someone who can lift your spirits and psych you up on your down days. Find someone who is on the same physical path and mental track that you are. Arnold would approach all the top bodybuilders he knew and ask if they were competing. Then he would ask them whether they wanted to win and how badly they wanted it. He would pick the guy with the most drive and the best positive attitude and ask him to be his partner.

How do you find a training partner? Ask, ask, ask. Ask family, ask friends, and ask coworkers. If you've exhausted asking people in your natural social network, then join a gym and introduce yourself to new people or put up classified ads in the gym, in the newspaper, or on the Internet.

Find a Mentor

The word "mentor" goes back to Greek mythology when Odysseus entrusted his friend Mentor with educating his son Telemachus when he left for the Trojan War. As in the Greek legend, a mentor is a teacher, guide, and trusted source of advice and wisdom. Mentors may be scholarly types or they may be a peer who has traveled your path, reached his destination, and is now giving back and sharing his knowledge gleaned from firsthand experience. In either case, they are wise old owls.

A mentor's primary purpose is educational support, because he's an expert in his field. This is not the person who holds your hand and coddles you emotionally. A mentor is the person who will teach you a skill, a science, an art, or a methodology. For how-to information, he is your go-to guy. In many cases, your ideal mentor is not only a teacher, but also someone you want to be like. Never choose a mentor based on knowledge alone. If you're going to crawl under somebody's wing, above all else, make sure they have character and integrity.

Call on Your Spiritual Community for Support

Spiritual advisers and religious communities are a major source of emotional support for millions of people across the world. For some, their spiritual community is the most important coping resource in their lives. Many people find it easier and more comfortable to trust and share with a friend from the church, synagogue, mosque, or temple than a friend from work. For people such as singles and childless married couples, their congregation may even serve as a type of surrogate family. Anyone with spiritual values and religious community ties might consider that this could be the most valuable social resource of all.

Join a Health Club

Joining a gym or health club can be your richest resource for new friends and partners. Ironically, it's the least pursued support strategy because many people don't feel comfortable in a gym. "I'd like to join a gym, but I have to get in shape first." The irony and comedy in that often heard reservation is obvious, but it's understandable because most people feel self-conscious about their weight and appearance.

Having worked as a health club manager for many years, I can say from experience that this fear of criticism is usually unwarranted. Most other people in the gym are self-conscious too. In fact, they're too busy thinking about themselves to pay much attention to you. I believe you're more likely to hear derogatory comments or experience discrimination on the street or in the workplace than you are in a health club.

I'm sure there are a few turkeys in every gym, but the predominant attitude I've seen among the gym veterans toward unfit or overweight people in the gym is respect. If other gym members notice at all, they'd be saying, "Good for them.

They took action." When the results start coming for newbies, they become the most respected members in the gym and role models to others.

Join an Internet Forum or Community

One place you can get all five types of support in one place is on the Internet. Web communities provide educational support through articles, audios, and videos with emotional support and personal accountability through e-mail, discussion forums, or chat rooms. Can this type of support really be worthwhile without face-to-face contact? Ultimately, only you can answer that, but the research says yes.

A study at Brown University published in the prestigious *Journal of the American Medical Association* confirmed that the Internet is a good way to deliver structured behavioral weight-loss programs. Lead researcher Deborah Tate, assistant professor of psychiatry and human behavior, reported on the results:

> **LOGGING ON MORE FREQUENTLY** was associated with better weight loss. It's especially important to look for new methods to help people with weight loss given that more than 64 percent of U.S. adults are overweight or obese. There are a lot of people who do not choose to attend face-to-face programs for any number of reasons, from embarrassment to schedule constraints. The Internet provides people with an alternative.

There are many forums and message boards on the Internet that are free, and I've seen people who don't even own a computer go to their local public library to log on. You can visit our support groups online at www.TheBodyFatSolution .com. Be picky about where you spend your time on the Web, and apply the same standards to your online friends as your personal friends.

When you consider joining a group, whether online or off, choose one where many of the members have already achieved their goals. Finding empathetic friends is important, but joining a group of people who are all at the same level as you is a great way to stay stuck there forever. To become more success-ful, surround yourself by, mingle with, and learn from successful people.

Bring Positive People into Your Life Through Books, Audios, Videos, and Websites

You have more freedom to change your environment than you might realize. You can invite positive people and energy into your own home through books, au-dios, websites, or videos. Within a few minutes you can make your environment more positive by placing motivational quotes, posters, or photos in your home or office.

I work by myself in my home office as a writer, but I'm never alone. One shelf is lined wall to wall with autographed photos of bodybuilding and fitness world champions. My office is filled with posters of athletes, inventors, and visionaries—people who did "the impossible." My library contains more than twenty-five hundred books.

Most people waste enormous amounts of time watching negative TV, read-ing trash, and surfing useless websites. You can use quality media to bring posi-tive energy into your life. It's all a matter of making the right choices.

Why People Don't Ask for Help

Support may be the one thing you need the most and the only thing missing in your health and fitness strategy. It takes courage to reach out, but if you don't, your social circle shrinks, your condition deteriorates, you withdraw even more, and you fall into a vicious cycle of isolation. Asking for help can be hard because we all want to feel strong and self-reliant. But asking for help when you need it is a sign of strength, not weakness.

Why don't people ask for help? It all boils down to fear. Fear of failure. Fear of criticism. Fear of judgment. Fear that others won't help. It's amazing what you can get if you have the courage to ask. Which kinds of support do you need? In-formation? Accountability? Comfort? A pat on the back? A swift kick in the rear end? Whatever you want and need, ask for it.

The R.E.A.C.H. Formula

You may have started reading this chapter feeling alone on your journey, not knowing where to turn for support. Now you have so many ideas for building a support circle, it might even seem overwhelming. That's why I've created a simple acronym that summarizes the lessons in this chapter, so you'll always remember how to find and use social support. It's called the R.E.A.C.H. formula.

REACH

Reach out to others. Don't wait for people to come to you. If you want support, ask for it. When the student is ready, the student must seek the teacher, not the other way around.

EXPRESS

Your friends and family are not mind readers. You have to communicate. Don't just ask for help, tell others how specifically they can help you and what type of support you need.

AVOID

Removing people from your life is a difficult decision, so never take it lightly. But if it comes to this point, remember that you're not losing friends, you're losing the people who weren't your friends.

CULTIVATE

Once you've reached out to others and expressed your feelings and needs to them, the relationship is just beginning. Relationships die on the vine if they're not nurtured.

HELP

A true social support system or mastermind group is a circle of receiving and giving. When someone gives you support, you need to give something back to them, or pay it forward to someone else.

Birds of a feather do flock together and you'll attract people to you based on the type of energy you put out. If you think new thoughts, speak new words, and take new actions, you'll attract new people into your life. But don't sit and wait for support to come to you. Go out and get it.

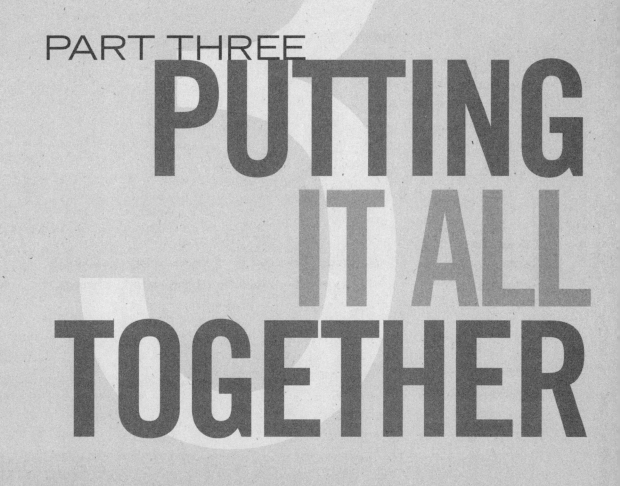

PART THREE

PUTTING IT ALL TOGETHER

CHAPTER TEN

Planning, Organizing, and Implementing

Focusing on Priorities, Putting It All Together, and Getting Started Right

THE main thing is to keep the main thing the main thing.

—STEPHEN COVEY, AUTHOR OF *THE 7 HABITS OF HIGHLY EFFECTIVE PEOPLE*

I f we gave your health and fitness habits a surprise examination today, what would be the prognosis? Be honest. Would your diet be in critical condition, in dire need of emergency treatment? Would your training program need a little patching up here and there? Do you even have a structured training program? How about your lifestyle? Is your body suffering the effects of late nights, alcohol use, or high levels of stress?

Regardless of your current physical condition, the absolute fastest way to improve your results is by prioritizing and planning. Your mission is to identify which areas in your life need immediate attention and then organize all your activities around those priorities. By following the formula you'll learn in this chapter, you could go from a complete standstill to full speed ahead and actually get better results in less time.

80-20: The Magic Formula for Achieving More by Doing Less

There's probably no better way to set priorities and increase your effectiveness than following the 80-20 rule. It was first discovered in 1897 by Vilfredo Pareto, an Italian economist who noticed a striking imbalance in the distribution of wealth. He found that 20 percent of the population had 80 percent of the money and assets.

In fitness, the 80-20 rule is counterintuitive. You might expect that every part of your training and nutrition would have approximately the same significance. Therefore, you usually treat each aspect equally. But the 80-20 rule applied to health and fitness says that 20 percent of your nutrition, training, and lifestyle habits will produce 80 percent of the changes in your body.

Understanding this principle can be disconcerting at first because you'll realize that most of what you were doing every day produced very little results. You may find yourself feeling like the proverbial gerbil on the wheel—lots of activity, but going nowhere fast. On the other hand, it's a profound revelation because it means that it's entirely possible to get more results from doing less.

When you understand how to use this to your advantage by implementing the rule, it's a life-changing paradigm shift. You realize that you don't have to sweat the small stuff, so in that sense, it's liberating. Your attitude becomes more relaxed and the whole endeavor is less stressful because you stop worrying about every tiny detail.

Applying the 80-20 rule is a process of identifying priorities and focusing more on those and less on everything else. It's not time management, it's activity management. It's the essence of working smart.

There are two ways to apply the 80-20 rule:

1. Spend more time and energy on the vital few (the 20 percent).
2. Spend less time and energy on the trivial many (the 80 percent).

The million-dollar question is, how do you know the difference between the important priorities and the trivial details? What are the 20 percent of activities that are producing the majority of your results?

Finding and Eliminating Bottlenecks

Think of the road to your perfect weight and ideal body as a huge multilane highway. Then imagine there's something blocking one or more of the lanes. As cars must merge to one side to squeeze through a narrow corridor, a choke point is created, causing traffic to back up for miles, slowing down your travel time or even bringing you to a complete stop. Anyone who has ever been stuck in traffic in Los Angeles or Chicago can relate to this because freeway bottlenecks in those cities cause 25 to 27 million hours of personal delay every year.

Needless delays also occur in your fitness journey because one or more major lanes of progress are blocked. Trainers often complain about their clients ruining all their hard work in the gym because even the best workout can't compensate for a lousy diet. One mistake in lifestyle such as sleep deprivation, poor choices in restaurants, or weekend bingeing can ruin an entire week of healthy eating. A single limiting belief, negative attitude, or emotional problem can sabotage *everything* you do.

Other common constraints include poor travel habits, skipping breakfast, emotional eating, binge drinking, poor exercise form, inefficient exercise programs, and inconsistency in any aspect of your nutrition or training.

Constraints can either be under your control (internal) or out of your control (external). Usually, you'll discover that the biggest constraints are internal. As Pogo said, "We have met the enemy and he is us." If you're not making progress toward your goal, there's almost always one major constraint blocking your path and you almost always have control over it. When you identify and remove it, your progress starts to flow through again at the maximum possible speed. Your body will start changing so fast it's almost scary.

A simple question or two can help flush out the major limiting constraint: What one obstacle is holding back your progress in every other area? What one fatal flaw has been preventing you from reaching your goal? Once you've pinned down the constraint, your priority is to pour the majority of your energy into resolving that one big issue.

The Hierarchy of Nutrition

One of the best ways to prioritize is by using the hierarchy approach. Abraham Maslow's hierarchy of needs, a psychological theory of motivation, was one of the most famous hierarchies. Illustrated as a pyramid, essential physiological needs such as food, water, and sleep formed the largest piece at the base, and esteem or self-actualization needs such as achievement and creativity were the smaller pieces stacked on top.

According to Maslow's hierarchy, if the most basic life needs aren't fulfilled, then they must become immediate priorities. Only when the essential survival needs have been met can the higher needs be pursued. This hierarchy concept is extremely helpful when you apply it to your training and nutrition.

More than forty nutrients are essential for your health, to provide energy, build or repair body tissues, and perform various bodily functions. For our purposes, we'll place them into five categories.

- **Energy intake.** Without adequate caloric intake, your body can't function at peak efficiency. A caloric deficit is an essential requirement for fat loss, but extreme and prolonged starvation diets decrease your metabolic rate. Caloric deprivation also makes it difficult to obtain all the other essentials.

Food is fuel and you have to fill up the gas tank every day if you want to get anywhere. Are you getting enough fuel?

- **Essential amino acids.** Protein is arguably the most important macronutrient when you're focusing on fat loss. Protein helps you hold on to lean tissue while you're in a caloric deficit and it even helps suppress your appetite. Essential amino acids, which are the building blocks of protein, can't be made by your body, so you must get them from your food. Are you eating a lean protein with each meal and meeting your daily protein requirements?

- **Essential fatty acids.** Essential fatty acids are vitally important for cardiovascular health and numerous body functions, including burning fat. Like essential aminos, the essential fatty acids can't be synthesized in your body and must be obtained from your food. Are you including healthy fat sources such as salmon every day?

- **Essential vitamins and minerals.** Vitamins and minerals are organic or inorganic compounds necessary for proper functioning of your body. They're essential because your body can't make them or can't make them in adequate quantities, so you must obtain them from your food. Fruits and vegetables are among the richest sources of these micronutrients. Are you eating them consistently every day?

- **Water.** Your body is mostly water. Water is so essential that without it you'd die in a matter of days. Even mild dehydration decreases physical performance. Adequate water intake is also necessary to burn fat optimally. Are you drinking enough water?

These are the essentials that must form the foundation of your pyramid. There are many minor details that can take your nutrition to a higher level. However, if you realize you're deficient in any of the foundational pieces, that's where your priorities must go. Refer back to Chapter Six and the ten nutrition rules to be sure your essential needs are met, above all else.

The Hierarchy of Training

The first essential of training is that you *are* training. Any training is better than no training. Many people spend hours and hours researching training techniques, but never get started. Many people, especially women, are hesitant to lift weights. But arguably, weight training is more important than aerobic training. Weight training can provide cardiovascular health benefits, but aerobics can't provide strength or muscular development benefits.

Your choice of exercises should also be prioritized using a hierarchy of importance. All exercises are not created equal. Always make the compound free-weight exercises such as squats, lunges, dead lifts, rows, and presses your first priority. The isolation exercises, such as curls, triceps extensions, and calf raises, are helpful but less important, and therefore, placed last in the workout. If you're ever pressed for time and need to shorten your workouts, drop these detail exercises first and always keep the major movements.

Most machines, with the exception of certain cable exercises, take lower priority than free weights. If your lower body workout consists of leg extensions, leg curls, inner thigh machine, and butt blaster machine, you need to put your priorities in order. Start squatting and deadlifting. You'll get more out of those two free weight exercises than all four of the machines combined.

Cardio is lower on the exercise hierarchy than weight training, but important nonetheless. The ideal program contains weight training and cardio training. Cardio provides its own unique health and fitness benefits and increases your total calories burned. As with weight training exercises, the type of cardio should also be prioritized.

Don't judge a cardio workout based on time alone. A twenty- to thirty-minute cardio workout could burn as many calories as a sixty-minute workout. The difference is intensity. If you're healthy, fit, and have no orthopedic or medical problems, then intense cardio goes higher on the hierarchy, especially if time efficiency is important to you.

Don't Waste Time on Minutiae

If 20 percent of your actions produce the majority of your results, then by definition 80 percent of your actions produce the minority of your results and are largely irrelevant. Worrying about minutiae is the fatal flaw in millions of people's fat-loss efforts.

For example, we have Mike the Macronutrient Micromanager, who slaves over spreadsheets for hours trying to tweak the ratios of protein, carbs, and fat to the tenth of a percentage point. Is it worth the trouble? Well, look at it this way: If you're on a starvation diet that leaves you deficient in protein, do you think it matters whether your paltry calorie intake is balanced perfectly to a 40-30-30 balance or whatever magical ratio you're trying to hit?

Then we have Annie Organic. She's forty pounds overweight and wants to know if she should eat organic fruits and vegetables to help her lose weight. Before I even start to explain any potential organic benefits such as avoiding pesticides or getting higher levels of micronutrients, I ask her how many fruits and vegetables she's eating now. I can't help but chuckle when she tells me she isn't eating any vegetables at all and only an occasional fruit, but she does have a problem kicking the daily candy habit. Wouldn't it make more sense to cut the sugar and eat more fruits and vegetables before worrying about organic versus traditional, or fresh versus frozen, or any of a dozen other details that don't matter if you're not eating any veggies in the first place?

Finally we have Pete the Pill Popper, who wants to know what fat burners to take—the whopper of all trivial pursuits. If you bought into the claims in most ads for diet pills, you'd come away believing you'd found the Holy Grail of weight loss. Ironically, in well-designed clinical research trials, at least 80 percent of supplements advertised for weight loss have never been proven to work for humans. Of the remaining 20 percent, 80 percent of those products don't do what the advertisements claim they'll do.

One nationally advertised fat-burner pill claimed that it would cure belly fat and melt away 20 percent of your body fat in three months. The research told a different story. Half the studies said it didn't work at all. The other half said it did work, but the results were barely significant. One double-blind, placebo-controlled clinical trial showed only one kilogram of weight loss in six months. Hundreds of thousands of people forked over $240 for a six-month supply of a supplement that produced trivial benefits, which easily might have been attributed to something else, even the placebo effect.

Don't the Details Matter Too?

Some people misinterpret the 80-20 rule to mean that almost everything they're doing is totally worthless. While that's not far from the truth at times, it's not entirely accurate. The 80 percent simply represents lower-value activities. If you're a competitive athlete, advanced trainee, or sophisticated dieter who has already mastered all the fundamentals and essentials, the details matter. A lot.

Another important success principle is known as the winning edge theory, which states that everything helps or hurts, nothing is neutral. This is especially important in sports, business, or competitive endeavors, where the slightest edge counts. Do details matter? Ask an Olympic swimmer for whom the difference between a gold and a silver medal was one-hundredth of a second. Ask the sprinter who placed fourth and missed the medals by a tenth of a second. If you're a professional athlete, then seemingly trivial details in practice, planning, and performance are the difference between making history and being an also-ran.

Everything matters. Everything counts. A small 100-calorie-per-day imbalance in energy—that's about four chocolate Kisses from the candy dish at work—could make you obese if you kept it up for a long enough period of time and everything else remained equal. The 80-20 rule doesn't imply that details don't matter. It says don't worry about the details until you've mastered the essentials. As Goethe said, "The things that matter the most must never be at the mercy of things that matter the least."

Always Have a Plan—Never Wing It

Imagine walking by a construction site and asking one of the workers, "Hey what are you guys building?" A worker replies, "I have no idea." I bet you've never heard such a thing because starting to build something without a plan would be pretty silly. But did you ever consider that it's every bit as silly to set foot in a gym, go grocery shopping, or even sit down at the dinner table without a goal and written blueprint for your nutrition and training?

I once heard a quote from motivational speaker Jim Rohn that changed my thinking forever. He said, "Never start your day until you finish it." At first it sounded like a riddle. How are you supposed to finish your day before you start it? Then the lightbulb went on and I realized that he was taking about planning before acting. The logical extensions are, never start your week until you've finished it, never start your month until you've finished it, and never start your year until you've finished it.

Action without planning is one of the biggest causes of failure. Planning takes serious thought and effort. It requires quiet, focused time with a pen and paper or computer, often with a coach or partner. Efficiency experts say that every minute spent in planning and preparation will save you ten minutes in execution.

When you apply this simple planning concept to your nutrition, training, and lifestyle, the results will dazzle you. Better results and more efficient use of time aren't the only benefits. Feeling unprepared or aimless creates anxiety and stress. That makes planning and preparation a superb stress reducer and confidence builder.

Planning and Organizing Around Priorities

Start every day, week, month, and year on paper. Always work from a list, plan, or schedule. Write a list of goals, a list of daily action steps, a daily schedule, a weekly schedule, a written meal plan, a written shopping list, and a written training plan. Create priority lists, not to-do lists. Priority lists focus on the vital few. To-do lists are usually cluttered with the trivial many.

The planning process begins with goal setting because all your activities must be organized around your high-priority goals and desired new lifestyle habits. Once your goals are in writing, apply 80-20 thinking. What is the one health, fitness, or body-weight goal that would make the biggest difference in your life if you achieved it in the next twelve weeks? Prioritize that goal by writing it on a card, carrying it with you everywhere you go, and reading it often.

Look at each of the five Body Fat Solution principles—mental training, cardio training, strength training, nutrition, and social support. In each of these categories, what is the one highest-priority goal or action step that will make the biggest difference in your life? Create your weekly schedule and daily action plan around these priorities.

Daily and Weekly Scheduling

Do you make appointments with your doctor? How about your dentist? Your accountant? Your hairstylist? How about your spouse or significant other—do you schedule a time and a day for dates? (Friendly tip: if you don't, exit visas are imminent.)

If you make appointments for everything else in your life, why would you leave your training to whatever scraps of time happen to be left over each day? Guess what? There never is any time left over. Mysteriously, your calendar will always fill up every day unless you set priorities and schedule blocks of time for what's most important to you.

You can start the planning process with nothing but a pen and a blank sheet of paper. I recommend investing in an appointment book or time planner. Scheduling each week in advance is easy because you already think and organize your life on a weekly basis. You'll also be setting body-weight and body-composition goals and charting your progress on a weekly basis, making seven days the perfect block of time for planning your training and nutrition.

I suggest writing your weekly training schedule into your time planner every

Sunday evening for the upcoming week. Then every night before going to bed, review your schedule and set daily goals and priorities for the next day. This way, your unconscious mind can absorb and integrate the information while you're sleeping. You'll hit the ground running in the morning with focus and direction.

At least one of your daily appointments will be your own workout. Write down the exact time you'll be training, the exercises or body parts you'll be working, and your goals for the session. Be specific. There's a huge difference between saying, "I'm going to work out tomorrow," and saying, "Tomorrow at seven a.m. sharp at Gold's Gym, I'm training hip-dominant lower body, horizontal push, horizontal pull, and lower abs, and I intend to break my personal dead lift record."

The Countdown Method

Another great planning technique is the "countdown calendar." I started using this method prior to my first bodybuilding competition. It worked so well for me, I've used it ever since and have recommended it to thousands of my clients who have also used it with tremendous success. Using a countdown, you'll get more focused and more motivated with each passing day as you see the deadline getting closer and closer.

If you don't have impending deadlines to give you a twinge in your stomach that screams, "Take action now, or else!" then you'll find it easier to say to yourself, "I have plenty of time, so one cheat meal or skipped workout doesn't matter." Then, when you realize you don't have time after all, you panic and engage in last-minute scrambling behaviors or you resort to extreme methods and dangerous quick fixes.

Here's how it works: get a wall or desk calendar—the type that shows each week stretching horizontally across the page with an open block of space for each day—or create your own eighty-four-day (twelve-week) chart on a computer in a word processor or spreadsheet.

Circle the goal deadline or competition date on the calendar and mark that as day zero. In each of the boxes, start counting backward from the present day:

T minus eighty-four days . . . T minus eighty-three days . . . T minus eighty-two days. This will program your unconscious mind to bring you in for a perfect landing on your deadline date, like an F-14 on an aircraft carrier.

Menu Planning

A written menu may be the single most important part of your plan. The advantage of working off a menu is that it's a proactive planning strategy. Many people keep food diaries or journals, and I don't discourage that at all because journals are a fantastic tool for education and accountability. However, journaling is not the same thing as working off a menu. With food journals, you eat something and then write it down. That's reactive. If you create a menu plan and then follow it, that's proactive.

A menu plan is literally your eating goal for the day. Starting your day without a menu plan is an invitation to wander off course at the slightest temptation or distraction. Working off a menu also means that you don't have to count your calories every day in real time. You only need to count your calories once when you create your menus. Then you simply follow the menu by weighing and measuring your food portions.

The ideal menu is one you create yourself using a template and general principles of meal construction, such as the ten nutrition rules you learned in Chapter Six. You can create menus on a blank sheet of paper and add up the calories by hand with a calculator, or you can use any of the commercial software programs available on the market today. Spreadsheets such as Microsoft Excel also work perfectly for menu planning and come already installed on many computers.

Organizing Your Kitchen

Your next step is to create a strategic plan for preparing your meals, including how you're going to eat at home, at work, in restaurants, and when traveling. The best place to start is in your own kitchen.

I've seen refrigerators filled with so much junk you'd need a GPS to navigate your way through them. Kitchen cupboards run a close second as the most cluttered place in the home. There's probably a lot of stuff in your kitchen that isn't supportive of your new health and fitness goals. Admit it. Then start Operation Kitchen Clean Sweep.

The biggest excuse I hear is, "I don't want to waste anything." We put that one to rest in Chapter Four, so don't even think about it. Throw it all out. Just because there's half a bag of potato chips in the cupboard doesn't mean you should eat them and then start your program after the bag is finished. If you're not going to drink sugary, high-calorie sodas anymore, then throw that two-liter cola bottle out. I don't care if you just bought it and haven't even cracked the seal. Pour it down the drain. It might not go to waste after all—it will probably clean some rust off your pipes.

If you have food stockpiled in the basement, garage, or some secret hideaway, clean those places out. Get rid of all the clutter, everywhere. If in doubt, throw it out. Once your kitchen is clean, keep it clean. If the junk's not there, you can't eat it.

Kitchen Essentials

Next, make sure you have all the essential kitchen appliances, utensils, cookware, and containers you'll need. In addition to the standard items found in every kitchen like a refrigerator, oven, and stove top, here are some of the essentials I have in my kitchen:

- grill pan
- sauté/omelet pan
- saucepans
- microwave oven
- rice cooker/steamer
- chopping knives
- microwave-safe cooking containers
- plastic food-storage containers
- resealable storage bags
- digital food scale
- measuring cups

Optional items include a blender and a George Foreman grill or some type of electric grill that can speed up your prep time by cooking chicken breasts and other lean meats quickly and in quantity. A rice cooker that doubles as a vegetable steamer is a godsend. Appliances that allow you to cook in bulk are wonderful time-savers.

Office Clean Sweep

Once your home is in order, it's time to clear out your office. Go through all your drawers and get rid of candy, pretzels, chips, and other low-nutrient-density, high-calorie-density snacks. You'll be bringing healthy snacks to work from now on. While you're at it, set up your work environment with little reminders to keep you focused on your goals. Post inspirational quotes and photos. Display your written goals prominently where you'll see them all day long.

What about that coworker temptress who drops off the doughnuts every morning? Tell her, "No, thank you," and ask her not to leave them anywhere in your sight or you'll throw them out. If she leaves them anyway, toss them and make sure she sees you do it. Remember, people hate to waste "perfectly good food." I guarantee she won't bring you doughnuts anymore. Works like a charm every time—especially if you dump them in the garbage can right on top of the pencil shavings and coffee grounds.

Planning your workday also includes deciding what you're going to eat for lunch. Don't leave home in the morning without knowing where you'll eat lunch and what you'll be having. If you think you won't have a wide enough range of options to make a healthy, low-calorie choice, then pack your own lunch. No excuses. The same goes for your midmorning and midafternoon snacks.

Planning Trips to the Supermarket

Dietitians estimate that 40 percent of supermarket purchases are made on impulse. Sometimes you'll have to inspect food labels at the store to make the better choice between two items, but all your major buying decisions should be made in advance. Follow my shopping tips below and you'll come out every time with low-calorie, high-nutrition food that moves you closer to your goals.

- **Always shop from a list.** Shopping lists are easy to create by using daily menu plans and adding up the supplies needed for a week's worth of menus. Once you have your list, stick with it. According to New York University nutrition professor Marion Nestle, 70 percent of shoppers bring lists into the supermarket, but only about 10 percent stick to them.
- **Don't shop hungry.** I'm sure you've heard this advice before, but do you follow it? Never shop on an empty stomach. Be mindful of your physical and emotional state as well. If you're tired or upset, you're more likely to grab junk food on impulse.
- **Shop quickly.** Did you know that supermarkets play down-tempo music to influence you to shop more slowly? It's true. If you linger longer, you buy more. Instead, with list in hand, see how fast you can zip through the store. It helps if you shop during off-peak hours when there are no crowds and shorter lines.
- **Do most of your shopping in the periphery of the store.** Eighty percent of the foods you'll want to eat on a regular basis can be found in the periphery of the store: fruits, vegetables, salads, potatoes, yams, lean meats, fish, seafood, dairy products, and eggs.
- **Beware of food product marketing.** In every square inch of the store, you're being marketed to constantly. Food companies pay for prime locations on the shelves. Appetite-stimulating colors such as red, orange, and yellow are used to draw your attention to snack foods. Stick to your plan and don't be taken in by marketing, including health and weight-loss claims.
- **Eat mostly foods with one ingredient and no label.** Eighty percent of the foods you eat daily will come without a label (think fruits and vegetables). If they have a label, they'll usually have only one ingredient, as in the case of lean meats, fish, eggs, or old-fashioned oatmeal.
- **Become an expert label reader.** Before eating anything in a box, can, or

package read the label carefully. Put it back if white flour or any form of refined sugars such as sucrose or high-fructose corn syrup are high on the list. Do the same if the ingredients include trans-fatty acids or chemicals with names you can't even pronounce. Also take note of the calories, serving size, and fiber amount.

- **Watch for label loopholes.** According to food labeling laws, if there's less than a half a gram of fat, the label can say "fat free." If there are fewer than five calories per serving, the label can say "zero calories." Food companies take advantage of these loopholes by shrinking their serving sizes. For example, a typical nonstick cooking spray will say "calorie free" on the label, but cooking spray is 100 percent oil. How do they get away with it? The serving size is a one-third-of-a-second spray.

- **Resist impulse purchases at the register.** Even as you're checking out, you're still being marketed to. Almost every checkout lane has candy and soda within arm's reach. If your store has a self-checkout minus the candy shelves, use that instead.

- **Shop for groceries online.** A study published in the *International Journal of Behavioral Nutrition and Physical Activity* found that people on fat-loss programs who ordered their groceries using online delivery services purchased 28 percent less calorie-dense foods than people who shopped in the supermarket.

Planning for Restaurant Eating

If there's one massive mistake that's more likely to sabotage your program than any other, it's making bad choices at restaurants. In study after study, eating frequently in restaurants correlates to higher body fat. It all makes sense when you look at how things have changed in the past several decades.

In 1955, Americans spent 19 percent of their food budget on meals prepared outside the home. Today that number has more than doubled to 41 percent. The number of people now overweight has more than doubled with it.

Obesity has tripled. According to the U.S. Department of Agriculture, $222 billion is spent every year at restaurants and $118 billion of that at fast-food restaurants.

The big problem: high-calorie meals, in part thanks to increasing portion sizes. Many typical restaurant meals contain 1,000 calories or more in the main course alone. If you include an appetizer and dessert, that could add 1,000 or more.

One slice of cheesecake for dessert can set you back 700 calories. Cheese nachos or fried mozzarella sticks have about 800 calories. The "normal" servings, that is. According to a report in *Men's Health* magazine, the worst nachos clocked in at 2,740 calories. A typical steak house prime rib or porterhouse could easily fall in the 1,200- to 1,500-calorie range. Imagine if you had appetizers, fries, dessert, and drinks with that.

The National Restaurant Association reports that the average person eats out 4.2 times per week. With that frequency, if you chose any of these "calorie bombs" each time you ate out, it would completely undermine every nutritious homemade meal you ate and everything you did in the gym all week long. Of course I realize that telling people they can't eat in restaurants won't make me very popular, so my more moderate suggestion is simply to keep restaurant eating to a minimum.

One of the characteristics I've discovered in the majority of lean people is that they prefer to keep tighter control over their nutritional intake by making most of their own meals. If the national average is four restaurant meals per week and you don't want an average person's body, then don't do what average people do. Do what lean people do. Keep restaurant dining to once or twice per week and make the right choices when you're there.

Regardless of how often you dine out, you have to educate yourself about the nutritional value of restaurant food and have a plan beforehand. For the sake of simplicity, I've condensed years of restaurant menu and food database research into one short checklist.

- Start with low-calorie salads instead of high-calorie appetizers.
- Avoid deep-fried foods such as French fries, onion rings, and calamari.
- Ask the wait staff not to leave the bread basket.
- Ask your server if you're not sure how something is prepared, especially about extra sauces, oil, butter, or other hidden calories.
- Look up menus and calorie information online and make a healthy choice in advance.
- If you don't know how many calories are in a dish, don't eat it.
- Choose grilled chicken or fish for lean protein.
- Choose lean sirloins or filets and get nine- to twelve-ounce cuts or smaller.
- Order steamed vegetables as side dishes.
- Order dry baked potatoes, sweet potatoes, or brown rice as sides or part of the main course.
- Order fresh fruit for dessert.
- Split a traditional dessert with a companion.
- Don't clean off your plate—take a doggie bag home with you.
- Eat only until you are 80 percent full. Never stuff yourself.
- Don't eat at buffets.

Planning Your Weekends

Unless your Saturdays and Sundays follow the same daily routine you follow on weekdays, it's important to plan your weekends in advance, especially your meals. A study conducted at Washington University and published in the journal *Obesity*, found that changes in schedule, meals, and lifestyle behaviors on weekends were enough to cause weight gain or slow down weight loss for the entire week. Many people can't figure out why they're not getting results when it seems like they put in so much effort all week long. The answer is that two days of indulgence can undo five days of work.

Planning for Holidays, Birthdays, and Special Occasions

Planning is also instrumental for navigating your way through holidays, birthdays, parties, and other special occasions. I believe that these are occasions where it's perfectly appropriate to relax and enjoy the food, family, and fun that are a part of these special times. However, this doesn't mean gorging yourself or throwing all caution to the wind.

Avoid all-or-none thinking. You don't have to choose between enjoying the holidays or staying lean and healthy—you can choose both. Holidays and other social events can very easily be worked into your 10 percent compliance rule. But when you commit to 90 percent compliance, honor your promise to yourself.

A common pattern, especially every November and December, is the "I'll start when" mind-set. For some reason, three holidays—Thanksgiving, Christmas, and New Year's—somehow translate into six weeks of nonstop dietary havoc. It's important to put this in proper perspective. It's really only three days you have to deal with. In fact, it's only a few meals. Enjoy the holiday food in moderation. The rest of the season it's training and nutritious eating as usual.

If you catch yourself saying, "I'll start when I get past the holidays," be careful, because that kind of thinking usually extends far beyond January 1, and you'll always be looking to start when conditions are just right. They never are.

Planning for Vacations and Travel

Just because you're traveling doesn't mean you can't follow your regular nutrition and training regimen. You spend so much time planning the flight, the car rental, the hotel, and other details of your trip, why not the training and nutrition? Here's the single most powerful technique I've ever used for travel fitness: nearly every time I travel, I set a goal to come home in better shape than when I left. Here's how to do it:

- **Get a hotel with a kitchen.** Many hotel chains offer rooms with a full kitchen. Or try short-term apartment or condo rentals. Search the Internet and you may be surprised at the type of lodging available and sometimes at better prices than hotels.

- **Go food shopping immediately after checking in.** After checking in, make a beeline to the local grocery store, shopping list in hand. Wherever you are in the world, if you have a kitchen and a well-stocked refrigerator, your meal planning and food preparation are not much different from when you're home.

- **Check the local restaurant menus in advance.** When you travel, it's likely that you'll have more restaurant meals than usual. Use all the restaurant-planning strategies you learned earlier and always think in advance about what you'll eat each time you dine out.

- **Cook portable foods and pack healthy snacks for drives, flights, and day trips.** For long flights and drives, nothing beats portable meals and snacks that you can carry with you. You can learn to make a variety of portable foods, including different types of oatmeal pancakes, healthy burgers, and healthy sandwiches. Frequent flying or driving is never an excuse for poor eating.

- **Write out your workout schedule in advance.** Keep using your time planner or schedule book even when you're away from home. Always work from a written plan.

- **Choose your training location in advance.** You can do body-weight exercises right in your hotel room. If you prefer, use the Internet to locate a gym prior to your trip. Call in advance and ask if there are daily or weekly rates. Ask if your hotel has a gym or an affiliation with a local health club. If you're a member of a gym in your local area, check to see if they are affiliated with other clubs around the country.

- **Make physical recreation part of your travel plans.** On one recent trip, I spent an entire day hiking in the hills of a beautiful national park. On another, I rented a bike and rode for miles along a beachside path. I've also noticed other people, many of them unfit, tooling around outside on those stand-up scooters. Which would you choose?

The Surefire Way to Implement New Habits and Lifestyle Changes

There's no way around it—to tackle a problem like body fat, which has so many causes, you must make changes in every area of your life. You have to eat better, train consistently, manage your emotions, change your thinking, get the support you need, and put it all together into a healthy lifestyle.

However, there's great power in prioritizing and concentrating on the single most important task at any given time. Many people try to do too much, too soon. The extremely motivated types may pull it off, but most people who dive in and make sweeping changes all at once merely scatter their focus, diffuse their efforts, and end up with a lower success rate in the long run.

A new habit usually takes about twenty-one consecutive days to form. If you focus on one primary goal or behavior change at a time, while keeping everything else in a holding pattern, you can form seventeen new habits in twelve months. With this approach, one year from now you will be such a changed person, you'll need a telescope to look back to the place where you started.

Find your biggest limiting constraint, follow the 80-20 rule, and use the hierarchy approach to choose the most logical places to start. Each person has unique strengths and weaknesses, so you'll have to carefully choose which areas you want to prioritize and focus on first. Here's one example of how the first six habit changes might play out.

1. Go to bed at ten to eleven p.m. sharp so you get seven to eight hours of quality sleep.
2. Take up yoga, meditation, or relaxation exercises to help reduce stress.
3. Start eating breakfast every day, which you may have skipped often. Try natural oatmeal, blueberries, and an egg-white scramble with one whole omega-3 egg.
4. Trade the leg "toning" exercises you were doing for free-weight squats and dead lifts.
5. Stop drinking alcohol or reduce to one to two drinks once or twice a week.

6. Stop drinking soda and switch to water or unsweetened green tea as your primary beverages.

Conclusion

What one change in your nutrition, exercise, or lifestyle habits would make the biggest positive difference in your body and your health? That's the question to ask yourself over and over again.

Keep in mind that your number one priority is usually not the easiest thing to do. It's easy to do the little stuff, and doing it makes you feel like you're achieving something, even though the returns are low. But never confuse activity with achievement. You could be busy, busy, busy, but if you're busy with minutiae, you're a gerbil on a wheel. The truth is, spending time on low-payoff activities is usually just procrastination or avoidance behavior. It lets you off the hook from doing what's difficult and necessary.

The 80-20 rule says that your best results will come from working hard on a small, selected number of highly productive actions. Unfavorable results occur when you spend too much time on the trivial many. Your task now is to identity the vital few actions, make them your priorities, then plan and organize your schedule and entire life around them.

One more thing: apply the 80-20 rule to this book. The truth is, about 20 percent of the information in this book will produce the majority of your results. I'm not sure which 20 percent that will be. But I do know that a few jewels of wisdom, carefully mined from these pages, could help you break through plateaus and achieve goals that have eluded you your entire life.

Keeping Score and Staying on Track

How to **Monitor** Your **Progress**, Make Yourself **Accountable**, and **Break Any Plateau**

CHAPTER ELEVEN

> **NO** battle plan ever survives first contact with the enemy.
>
> **—MILITARY AXIOM**

Management consultant and business author Ken Blanchard once said, "Feedback is the breakfast of champions." That's great advice, and it's just as true for managing your own body as it is for managing a company.

The formula for success is simple: first, you set a specific goal with a deadline. Second, you devise an action plan or strategy for achieving your goal.

243

Third, as soon as you have a plan in writing, you launch into action, whether you think you're ready or not.

That brings us to the fourth step—getting feedback and adjusting your approach according to your results. It's a vitally important step that too many people forget or avoid.

Staying on Track with Performance Feedback

Feedback means measuring your results at frequent intervals to see if your action plan is working and to make sure you're on the right track. Put another way, it means you have to "keep score."

Many weeks, months, and even years are wasted because people fail to make themselves accountable for their actions and their results. Millions of people are confused by conflicting information about nutrition and weight loss, but all their questions would be answered simply by measuring their progress. A single measurement is worth a thousand opinions.

Many people avoid measuring progress and holding themselves accountable because honest feedback can be painful. But if you avoid getting feedback to avoid feeling hurt and disappointed, what you're really doing is staying inside your comfort zone. You're hiding from the fact that you're falling short of your potential and could be doing a lot better.

Some people fail to get the feedback they need because they don't know how to measure it systematically or they don't know what to measure. We are a weight-conscious society, but weight is not the only feedback you need. If you were solid muscle and nothing on your body jiggled (unless it was supposed to), would you care how much you weighed?

Body weight includes fat, muscles, bones, internal organs, and even the contents of your digestive system. Your body is also 70 percent water, which means that shifts in hydration can affect the scale dramatically, literally overnight. The scale is an important and helpful tool for measuring progress, but the scale can also fool you.

Body composition refers to what percentage of your total body mass is made up of muscle versus fat. When food or calorie restriction are taken to an extreme, and especially without weight training, it's entirely possible to lose more muscle than fat.

A body fat test lets you separate your total body weight into lean tissue versus fat tissue instead of measuring only body weight. This gives you a much clearer picture of the effects your nutrition and training are having on your body.

How to Measure Your Body Fat

There are many ways to measure your body fat, but not all of them are suitable for repeated, personal use. For example, underwater weighing, also known as hydrostatic testing, has been called the gold standard because of its high accuracy. However, hydrostatic testing is not very practical. Who wants to go to get dunked every week while suspended from an oversized grocery scale?

Magnetic resonance imaging (MRI) and dual energy X-ray absorptiometry (DEXA) are two of the most accurate high-tech methods for body composition testing. The problem is these tests are usually only performed in hospitals or research facilities, so they're too inaccessible or expensive for weekly use.

If you ever get a chance to get tested by DEXA or hydrostatic weighing, I'd recommend it. However, for our purposes, you need a method that's simple, practical, accessible, and inexpensive. That's where skinfold testing comes in.

A device called a skinfold caliper is used to pinch a fold of skin and fat and measure the thickness in millimeters. Your skinfolds are then translated into a body-fat percentage estimate using special regression equations (detailed instructions and conversion charts usually come with the calipers).

One option is to have a trainer or fitness professional measure your body fat if this service is available at your local health club. Sometimes there's a small fee, although some clubs offer the testing for free to their members. Try to find a trainer who has a lot of experience doing these tests because caliper testing is only as accurate as the person doing the pinching.

Another choice is an inexpensive plastic skinfold caliper. One of the most popular models is the Accu-Measure, which was designed specifically for home self-testing. The Accu-Measure requires you to pinch a skinfold at only one location—your iliac crest (hip bone). If you have a friend or partner willing to help, you can use an inexpensive plastic skinfold caliper such as the Slim Guide model for a multisite pinch test. Generally, if you use a body fat test that measures three or four skinfold sites, you get a more accurate body fat estimate.

There's a lot to be said for the accountability factor of having a coach or trainer measure you every week. However, the privacy factor of home testing is also nice because you may prefer not to have a stranger groping your fat rolls every week. Once you start getting leaner, though, you may surprise yourself when one day you're proud to have someone "pinch you," because there's nothing there but thin skin on top of solid muscle.

What About Body Fat Scales?

One disadvantage of caliper testing is that if you're extremely overweight, it's sometimes difficult to take the measurements. The accuracy of skinfold tests tends to decrease when body fat levels are very high.

An alternative method for private home testing is the "body fat scale." Body fat scales are based on bioelectrical impedance analysis technology (BIA). You step on it like a regular scale, and it not only displays your weight on the digital readout, but also your body fat percentage.

Whereas underwater weighing measures body fat by a method based on the fact that fat floats and muscle sinks, the BIA test measures it by a method involving electrical conductivity. Muscle has high water content and is highly conductive. Fat has lower water content and is not highly conductive.

When you step on the scale, a current is passed through your lower body to measure your tissue's resistance to electricity. Don't worry, you don't feel anything because it's a low-amperage current (although I've had a few "trouble" clients I wouldn't have minded giving a shock at times). BIA hand-gripper devices use the same impedance technology as the scales; they simply pass the current through your upper body only.

Because an electrical conductivity test is influenced by body water, anything that affects your water balance, such as alcohol, caffeine, diuretics, exercise, heat, and even the time of day, can skew your results. To get accurate and consistent readings, it's important to follow the instructions that come with the scale and perform the test under the same conditions every time.

Some research has validated body-fat-testing scales, but the research is mixed and so is user feedback. Fluctuations in measurements can occur depending on the time of day and test conditions. Some people report a 5 percent difference between morning and night. Others say that they can step on the scale once, then step on it again a minute later and get a totally different reading—like 2 or 3 percent lower.

I prefer skinfold caliper testing, but any method you can use frequently with consistent readings will work. Whichever method you choose, stick with it. Using two different methods will often give you two different results, which only makes tracking your progress more difficult.

What's an Ideal Level of Body Fat?

High body fat levels have been linked to more than thirty health problems, including diabetes, high blood pressure, cardiovascular disease, cancer, and osteoarthritis. Being categorized as clinically obese means that body fat is so high that health problems become a concern. Men are considered clinically obese at 30 percent, while women are clinically obese at 35 percent body fat.

Competitive bodybuilders and endurance athletes such as marathon runners have been known to reach body fat levels as low as 3–4 percent in men and 8–9 percent in women. Being very lean is undoubtedly healthier than being obese. Trying to maintain extremely low body fat levels for too long, however, may by unhealthy and unrealistic. This is particularly true for women. At extremely low body fat levels, women may begin having problems with estrogen production. Menstrual cycles and reproductive systems become disrupted and bone density may decrease, putting them at higher risk of osteoporosis as they grow older.

It's impossible for your body fat to drop to zero, since some fat is necessary for normal body functioning. This is called "essential fat" and it's required for energy storage, protection of organs, and insulation against heat loss. Essential fat is found in the nerves, brain, bone marrow, liver, heart, and in nearly all the other glands and organs of the body. In women, this fat also includes sex-related fat deposits, such as breast tissue and uterus. Essential body fat is at least 2–3 percent for men and 7–9 percent for women.

If your goal is to get leaner, then your ideal level of body fat is a level lower than it was last week. Personal improvement should be your goal, more so than hitting a certain number. Having very low body fat is nice for bragging rights, but don't obsess over the numbers. See those numbers for what they really are: a way to quantify your results and get feedback on your progress.

Having made that point, here are some averages and ideals to give you an idea where you stand and where you should be aiming. The average adult woman has about 23 percent body fat and the average man about 17 percent. The numbers increase slightly with age. The average twenty-year-old male college student has about 15 percent body fat. The average sedentary middle-aged-male has 20 percent body fat or more.

Body fat of 25 percent would still place a female in the "average" category, but averages aren't necessarily ideal. An ideal percentage of body fat for a nonathlete is around 10–14 percent for men and 16–20 percent for women. At "good" body fat levels, you'll be lean enough to start showing some muscle definition. At "excellent" body fat levels, you'll be nicely defined and every area will be firm and tight. When will you see those coveted "six-pack abs"? Most men

Body Fat Rating Scale

	men	women
Extremely lean ("ripped")	3–6%	9–12%
Very lean (excellent)	< 9%	<15%
Lean (good)	10–14%	16–20%
Average (fair)	15–19%	21–25%
Below average (poor)	20–25%	26–30%
Major improvement needed (very poor)	26–30%+	31–40%+

will start to see their abs when they hit the single digits. Women start to see that kind of muscle definition when they reach the midteens.

How to Set a Weekly Body Fat Goal

I recommend setting a fat reduction goal of about a half a percent per week. If your body fat measured 24.6 percent on Day One of Week One, then 24.1 percent would be your goal for the end of that seven-day period. That will be an impressive 6 percent drop in your body fat if you keep that up over twelve weeks.

If you're more ambitious and you want to shed body fat even faster, it's certainly possible. I've seen many people drop 0.6 percent or 0.7 percent body fat per week if they worked very hard, usually doing four to six cardio sessions per week combined with excellent dietary compliance. I've even seen people shed 0.8 percent, 0.9 percent, even 1.0 percent per week, but those were almost always temporary spikes in progress.

Anything over a half a percent per week should be considered above-average progress. And remember, achieving above-average results will require above-average efforts.

Body Mass Index and the "Skinny Fat" Syndrome

One of the most popular ways to judge whether you're overweight or obese is the body mass index (BMI). BMI is calculated by dividing your weight in kilograms by your height in meters squared. You're considered underweight if your body mass index is less than 18.5. Normal weight is a body mass index of 18.5 to 24. If your BMI is above 25 you are overweight, above 30 and you are obese, or so they say.

The problem with BMI is that it doesn't tell you anything about your body composition. What if you weigh more than average and you're mostly solid muscle? For example, Tim, one of my inner-circle members, was 235 pounds at six feet tall.

"When I was in the Army, I had to be body fat tested all the time to make sure I met military standards, because according to my BMI of 31.9, I was obese," he explained. "Of course, I was far from obese. I was in a unit where the physical training was very intense and my body fat measured twelve to thirteen percent. Being built like a linebacker, the BMI will probably always tell me I am obese, which is why I ignore it completely."

There's another dark side to BMI, as well. You could have a low BMI but high body fat. In a study conducted at St. Luke's Roosevelt Hospital in New York, researchers found a strong correlation between body fat percentage and BMI, but there were also many exceptions. One fifty-year-old woman had a normal BMI of 23.3, but her body fat measured 30 percent. Scientists call this normal weight obesity. In the common vernacular, it's known as "skinny fat."

These two examples should open your eyes to the big problem we have with the way our society approaches so-called ideal body weights. Most people are so fixated only on the pounds of body weight and the outward appearance of "thinness," they're not paying attention to health, strength, and body composition. These are the measures of success that count the most, so most of your goals and progress tracking should revolve around them.

Waist and Other Body Circumference Measurements

Your waist measurement doesn't tell you your exact body fat percentage or lean body mass, but there is a high correlation between waist measurement and body fat that makes it a valuable number to track. If your waist is going down, you can be almost certain that your body fat percentage is going down.

Waist girth also reveals different aspects of body composition and disease risk. The size of your belly reflects not only the subcutaneous fat that's below your skin, but also the deeper intra-abdominal, or "visceral," fat. Also known as central obesity, a high waist measurement of thirty-five inches or more for women and forty inches or more for men is a risk factor for metabolic syndrome, cardiovascular disease, type 2 diabetes, and cancer. Thigh fat may be annoying, triceps flab can be unsightly, but abdominal fat can be deadly.

You may find taking other body measurements to be helpful. Measuring your hips, thighs, arms, or any other circumference is an option. Keep in mind, however, that losing inches is not always the same as losing fat. Losing inches could reflect the loss of water. Gaining inches could mean an increase in muscle. No change could indicate a loss in fat and a gain in muscle at the same time.

Why You Should Weigh Yourself Often

Have you ever been told by a weight-loss expert to throw away your scales? Most people have because it's common advice today. Surprisingly, almost all the studies on the subject say the opposite: self-monitoring behaviors of all kinds, including counting calories, journaling food intake, logging your workouts, measuring your body fat, and, yes, weighing yourself, help increase adherence and improve results.

Research has also concluded that people who monitor progress and weigh themselves frequently improve weight maintenance and avoid weight regain or weight cycling as compared to people who don't weigh themselves at all.

Your body weight can jump quickly when there are sudden changes in your lifestyle or environment, but usually weight gain sneaks up on you. Body fat "creeps" when it's not checked. Folks who don't monitor weight or body composition seem to wake up one morning and notice that they "suddenly" got fat. Of course, what really happened is that tiny increases in fat and waistline went unchecked and, therefore, unnoticed over a long time period.

Weigh yourself often, at least once a week, but pay the most attention to your weight trend over time. If your weight spikes overnight, don't worry too much about that. If your weight is steadily climbing from week to week, then inside your mind, there should be sirens blaring, alarms going off, and red lights flashing everywhere. Warning, warning, danger, danger.

Do not tolerate weight creep. When you see it happening, nip it in the bud. Buckle down on your compliance or change your strategy immediately.

By the way, people who have to wear well-tailored suits or tight-fitting clothes have a feedback mechanism for checking themselves every day. Those who wear baggy clothes or elastic waistbands and who don't weigh themselves tend to be more susceptible to the weight creep. If you wear loose, baggy clothing most of the time, then it's not a bad idea to have a pair of "lean jeans" that you try on regularly to see how they're fitting.

If you understand statistics, then you know that daily weighing can be extremely helpful, as long as you use that daily weight data to look at the weight trend and you don't obsess over short-term fluctuations. Your weight fluctuates not only on a daily basis, but even on a within-day basis, sometimes by several pounds. Your weight fluctuates based on changes in body water, the contents of your digestive system, the levels of glycogen in your muscles (stored carbohydrates), and, for females, the time of the month.

Like looking at stock market charts, the short-term peaks and valleys shouldn't alarm you. People who invest wisely and hold almost always win in the long term compared to people who panic during brief market fluctuations or jump on random tips. It's the same with your body. It's a positive trend over time that should interest you the most. During the fat-loss phase, body fat and body weight should be heading downward in a steady trend and lean body mass should be holding relatively stable or increasing slightly.

If you weigh yourself daily, you can log your weight into a spreadsheet and then convert your progress into a graph with the date on the horizontal axis and weight/body composition on the vertical axis. You can even keep track of your trend with a seven-day moving average if you choose, which smoothes out the fluctuations, or "noise." I've noticed that it's the analytical types, such as accountants and engineers, who like to see as much data as possible. If that's not your style, then don't sweat it. Just log in your weight once a week.

Regardless of your weighing frequency, consistency is vital. To get the most accurate data possible, do your best to duplicate the weigh-in conditions every time: fed or fasted, clothed or not clothed, bladder empty or full, pre- or post-workout, morning or evening, high-carb or low-carb day, and so on. For example, if you opt for once a week, then make your official weigh-in every Monday first thing in the morning after a bathroom visit and before eating or exercising.

Your First Week: Finding Your Baseline

If you're traveling in an unfamiliar city and don't know where you are, you would describe that as being "lost." If you're lost, you can't plot a route to where you want to go. You have to get your bearings first. That's why the first step is always assessment, which means finding out where you are now and establishing a baseline.

In athletics, physical assessments often include a huge battery of physiological and performance tests. For you, the assessments will be much simpler. On the first day you start this program, you're going to take an inventory of what kind of shape you're in. I know this part may be difficult, but everyone starts somewhere and you need to know where your somewhere is in order to plot your course properly.

Measure anything you want to improve. The more things you measure and record, the better. You might even want to work in conjunction with your doctor to keep track of important health indicators. It's so rewarding and motivating to watch your blood pressure, triglycerides, and cholesterol drop as your weight and body fat drop. Always remember, it's not just about the body-fat percentage and the pursuit of six-pack abs. Your ultimate goal is to be lean and healthy, not just lean.

Your Weekly Progress Chart

I strongly encourage you to measure and record your body composition weekly. Your weekly progress chart is how you keep score. It's your report card. You could take measurements less frequently, but the more often you measure, the more feedback you'll get, and the less time you'll have wasted if you find that you drifted off course.

Once you've done your initial Week One assessments, repeat the process weekly on your official weights and measures day. I recommend Mondays because that's the start of a new week and it helps keep you more honest on the weekends, when you may be more likely to slip off track.

You can design your own chart to record your progress. The important information that belongs on every progress chart is as follows:

- date
- body weight
- body fat percentage
- pounds of body fat
- pounds of lean body mass
- waist circumference

Once you know your weight and body-fat percentage, it's easy to calculate your pounds of fat and pounds of muscle. For example, if you weigh two hundred pounds and you have 10 percent body fat, then you have twenty pounds of fat (10 percent of 200 = 20). That means you have a lean body mass of 180 pounds. With this data on your chart, you can get the clearest picture of how your exercise and nutrition programs are really affecting your body.

If you notice that your lean body mass is decreasing, you'll need to take corrective measures quickly. This includes checking for adequate protein intake, making sure your caloric intake isn't too low, keeping up with your weight training program diligently, and making sure your lifestyle is in order regarding sleep, stress, and overall recovery.

Photos

Photographs are fabulous tools for documenting your progress, even though they're visual feedback and they don't give you any numbers to work with. Everyone has a certain degree of distorted self-image in the way they see themselves in the mirror and in their own minds. But there's something different about photographs. The photos don't lie.

The benefits of photographs can go far beyond progress charting. Sometimes seeing a photograph of yourself is the pivotal event that triggers a turn-around in your lifestyle. Aimee, one of my inner-circle members, related her experience in our group forum:

> **I HAD BLOWN UP TO** one hundred fifty pounds and I'm only five feet tall, so that was the heaviest I've ever been in my life. Then I had my body fat measured and was shocked to learn that it was 35 percent. But it wasn't until I was flipping through some pictures that it hit me and I realized for the first time what I really looked like to other people. I said, how did this happen? Seeing a picture of me was the experience that made me start Tom's program, join the gym, and that's when I really started to change. Today I weigh 106 pounds and I wear a size zero.

Take out the most recent pictures of yourself and have a good look at them. If you don't have any current photos, take some pictures right now from every angle. Those will be your "before" photos. It's up to you whether you post them on a website or share them with anyone else, but at least do this for yourself.

Weekly photos are invaluable as a progress charting tool. I know a lot of people who didn't want to get in front of the camera when they started, but I know even more people who regretted not taking "before" photos after they had reached their ideal weight and body fat goals.

The Power of Accountability

Accountability is one of the greatest benefits of tracking your results by the numbers. Internal accountability is becoming answerable for your actions and results by measuring and recording them. External accountability is when you report those actions and results to someone else or someone else measures and tracks them for you.

In business, there's a saying, "If you can't measure it, you can't manage it." Good managers have found that personal productivity and company profitability can be increased many times over by measuring and tracking everything. This often means having employees use numerous checklists, sales reports, and even hourly diaries showing how they spend their time. Those lists and diaries are turned in and inspected by the boss.

Every team member knows their results are being monitored and they'll be graded on performance. This creates a massive amount of leverage. A good accountability system is so powerful that business owners don't even have to be in the store all the time, they simply need devices in place for measuring the activity and output of their team.

It's the same with your nutrition and training. Performance improves when performance is measured and reported. As a personal trainer and fitness coach, accountability has always been something I've taken seriously and built into every program I've ever created. When my clients knew they were going to be weighed and measured every week, they worked harder during the week in anticipation of the test day. Progress charts were held sacred. Like a bad grade on a report card, no one wanted a blemish on their weekly progress chart.

My local coaching clients met with me in person where they would step on the scale in front of me and I took their body fat measurement with calipers. But it was amazing to see how effective these twelve-week coaching programs were, even when I was working long-distance with clients on the other side of the world.

Every Monday morning—accountability day—my long-distance clients would e-mail or fax me their progress charts. If they had unfavorable results the previous week, I would be asking for their eating and training journals, as well. If they knew I was going to be looking through their journal like a professor at a term paper, I knew they would stick with the program better.

Who are you accountable to? Who do you answer to? Ask yourself these questions every day. If the answer is no one, then find someone quickly.

Accountability on the Internet

Having in-person support provides benefits you can't get any other way. Accountability, however, is so powerful that even without face-to-face contact, the results can be astonishing. Accountability doesn't even have to be provided by a professional coach or personal trainer. All you have to do is be accountable to yourself, first by tracking all your results, then showing your results to someone else.

If you want to increase your motivation and improve your results, then you can use the Internet to share your results with anyone, anywhere in the world. Today, there are thousands of people in every country using blogs as electronic fitness journals and accountability tools.

A blog, which is short for Web log, is a like an online journal that you can create in just minutes, even if you have no clue how to build a website. If you have access to a computer and you can type, then you can blog. You can build a blog on your own website domain for minimal cost, or use a free blog service such as blogger.com, which is now owned by the search-engine giant Google.

With blogs, discussion forums, and online social networking groups, it's easier than ever to hold yourself accountable. In many discussion groups, there are forums designated for progress journals and photo galleries where you can post your "before," "during," and "after" photos. Some websites provide a place where you can keep your nutrition journal online, and they may even do all the calorie and macronutrient calculations for you.

You can join a small group where you feel comfortable sharing your progress or you can post publicly where the whole world can follow your fitness journey.

Training Journals

Training journals serve a dual purpose, since they're important progress-charting tools as well as accountability devices. Unless you have a photographic memory, there's no way you can keep track of the sets, reps, and weights you used in every workout for months and years on end. By opening up your journal, you can see your previous workout and your previous best efforts and plan your upcoming workouts accordingly.

A good training journal will contain, at the very least, the date, the name of the exercises performed, the sets, reps, and poundage lifted. You can be much more detailed and creative if you feel the need.

A journal can also include a record of lifestyle factors, such as your hours of sleep, quality of sleep, stress levels, energy levels, and recovery. Journaling these types of factors and quantifying them on a rating scale such as 1 to 10 can help raise your accountability and trace the correlations between your methods and your results. Your journal can also include a place for all your personal records (PRs). Some people even create a separate PR journal, or "victory journal."

PR journals are terrific motivators. Always striving to break your own personal records gives you a whole new set of goals to aim for. It makes your training fun, exciting, and challenging. Competing against your own personal bests is the ultimate type of competition. What's most important is not whether you're better than someone else, but that you're better than the you of yesterday.

Nutrition Journals

Nutrition journals can be kept in writing, or electronically using websites, software, or handheld devices. The first time you do it, it can be quite a wake-up call. You almost never realize how much you're eating until you see it on paper and add it all up.

Keeping a real-time nutrition journal is optional if you work off a menu, but a three-day nutrition recall can be a valuable part of the initial assessment process. Think back over the last three days and write down everything you ate. Once you've got the food items listed, tally up your calories. The usual verdict is that you've been guilty of eating a lot more calories than you thought you were.

Nutrition journals are outstanding accountability tools. When you have a written record of your daily food intake and you share it online or you turn it in to a coach or accountability partner, you'll be amazed at how your behavior changes.

In fact, it has always been a challenge for nutritionists to get accurate dietary records because the moment that nutrition is tracked, people start to alter their eating behaviors. This "observer effect" comes into play because the journaling makes you more aware of what you're eating, and no one likes to admit their nutritional mistakes.

Dealing with Ups and Downs

It's bound to happen sooner or later: you either hit a plateau or you have a bad week where you don't meet your compliance rule. Success isn't always smooth sailing all the way. Usually, you make progress in spurts, you hit plateaus, which must be broken, and face obstacles that must be overcome.

The first step in dealing with these inevitable ups and downs is to accept that they're going to happen and prepare yourself to handle them physically and mentally. One of the ultimate emotional skills you can develop is the ability to stay calm and optimistic in the face of negative results or unexpected events.

As soon as the going gets tough, most people buckle. Some people will even abandon their biggest goals and dreams just because the first thing they try doesn't work. Other people have ferocious persistence and never let go of their goals. They're like a bulldog that refuses to release its teeth-hold on a bone. The harder you try to pull it out of his mouth, the more it growls and chomps down harder.

Dr. Martin Seligman, a professor of psychology at the University of Pennsylvania, did some amazing research on the differences between people who quit and people who persist. The answer was in what he referred to as "explanatory style," which is the way we explain or interpret bad events or failures.

People who habitually give up have an explanatory style of permanence. They hit a plateau in their diet and explain it by saying, "Diets never work," or "I have bad genetics, so I'll always be fat." These explanations imply a permanent and pervasive situation. Other people hit a plateau and explain it by saying, "I ate too much fast food this week," or "I missed a couple of workouts." These explanations imply that the circumstances are temporary and under your control.

The people who see obstacles as temporary are the ones who never quit. If you have a bad day, mess up a meal, or miss a workout, just tell yourself, "It happens. This too shall pass." Remind yourself it was just one meal. It was just one workout. It was just one day. Tomorrow is a new day.

Fat-Loss Plateaus and Why They Happen

You might think that if you planned your nutrition and training well enough and took action consistently enough, then you'd never hit a plateau. Unfortunately, your biology has its own plans.

Your body not only adapts quickly to training programs, it also adapts to a reduced-calorie intake to help regulate and stabilize your body weight. The result is that your weight loss will automatically slow down over time, even if you don't change a thing in your strategy. If you do inadvertently make a nutrition or training mistake, your fat loss can stall completely.

The knee-jerk reaction for most people is to blame the plateau on something out of their control, usually a slow metabolism, bad genes, or a thyroid problem. But to get past a plateau, you need to acknowledge what a plateau really is. If you were losing weight but then your progress stalled, there's only one thing that can mean: you were in a calorie deficit, but you're no longer in a calorie deficit. There are five major reasons why this happens.

1. Your metabolic rate slows down. Scientists call it "adaptive thermogenesis." The more popular term is "starvation mode." Your body interprets a severe and prolonged calorie shortage as famine, so it automatically decreases your metabolic rate in order to conserve energy. This decrease in metabolism from calorie restriction is not enough to cause a plateau, but it's enough to slow down your progress so your actual weight loss doesn't match what you would predict on paper.

2. After people lose a lot of weight, they tend to keep eating the same way they were eating when they were heavier. But when you're a smaller person, you don't need as many calories.

Here's an example: Kevin is a moderately active forty-year-old male, 5 feet 8 inches tall, and 235 pounds. With these stats, he would require about 3,200 calories per day to maintain his weight. Using a conservative calorie deficit of

20 percent below maintenance level, he would want to consume 2,600 calories per day to lose weight.

Suppose Kevin successfully drops fifty pounds and becomes a lean 185-pounder, but he still wants to cut the last ten pounds so he can finally see his abs. If you recalculate his calorie needs at his new body weight, all else being equal, he now only needs about 2,800 calories to maintain his smaller body. If he keeps eating 2,600 calories per day, he is barely in a calorie deficit anymore. If he forgets to report one little 200-calorie snack, there's his "unexplainable" plateau. To drop the last ten pounds, he has to either eat less or exercise more to accommodate his new body size and get the calorie deficit back.

3. When you move your new, smaller body, you're not burning as many calories. If you don't believe it, then take this simple test: strap on a forty-pound weighted vest or backpack and go hike up a steep hill. Obviously, if you're lugging around extra weight, you're burning more calories. The reverse is also true: after you lose weight, you burn fewer calories to move your lighter body.

4. Most people either cheat on their diets or they forget to record part of their food intake, and they do it more often at the tail end of a diet when appetite is turned up a notch. Studies have showed underreporting calorie intake as much as 50 percent is common. In other words, you might swear you're only eating 2,000 calories per day, and you can't figure out why you're stuck at a plateau. In reality, you gave in to the hunger and underestimated your food intake. You're really eating 3,000 calories a day, which doesn't give you any caloric deficit.

5. There is inconsistency over time. Kim is a female with a maintenance level of 2,100 calories per day. Suppose Kim eats 1,600 calories per day Monday through Thursday. Four for four. She's right on target for a one pound per week weight loss. But then on Friday, Kim goes out to dinner and inadvertently finishes her day at 2,500 calories. On Saturday she attends a wedding and by the time the reception is over, she has topped 2,700 calories thanks to dinner, cake, and champagne. On Sunday, she struggles to get back on track, but ends up even at 2,100 calories.

Add it all up and you get 13,700 calories for the week. That's 1,957 calories per day on average. Over the entire seven-day period, Kim barely had a calorie deficit and her body fat loss will be almost immeasurable. At that rate, it would take her twenty-three days to lose one pound of fat. Kim doesn't realize how inconsistent she's been with her nutrition, so she grumbles about her "slow metabolism" and starts searching for the next diet "breakthrough."

What really happened is she only remembered the four good days that she followed her program perfectly and she didn't realize how much damage she did on the weekend. This is also known as "remembering the hits and forgetting the misses." Consistency is one of the major keys to success and it's a virtue that many people need a lot of work on.

Why the Last Ten Pounds Are So Hard to Lose

The last ten pounds are almost always a lot harder to lose than the first ten. That's why a truly ripped set of six-pack abs is such a rare sight.

If you have difficulty getting the weight loss started or if you get stuck early on, you can almost always bet that you have some kind of compliance, underreporting, or inconsistency issue. Double-check your calorie intake closely, especially on weekends and when you eat at restaurants. Start keeping a journal and be ruthlessly honest with yourself about how well you're following your plan.

In the later stages of your diet, however, some of the difficulty you might experience with the last few pounds has biological origins. Yes, it's true. In some cases, it's not your fault that fat loss slows down. It's only your fault if it stays that way because you fail to make the adjustments and kick-start your progress again.

Once you start to get very lean, or if you're still carrying a lot of fat but you've been in a caloric deficit for a long time, your body sounds the starvation alarm. If you think about it from a survival-of-the-species point of view, it's not beneficial to have very low body fat. That's why the leaner you get and the longer you've been dieting, the more your body fights to hold on to whatever fat is left.

With prolonged and severe dieting, your metabolism decreases more sharply and does everything it can to get you off your diet. A decrease in leptin levels is one reason this happens. Also known as the antistarvation hormone, leptin is a hormone, produced primarily in your fat cells, that tells your brain how the fuel supplies are doing. If fat stores are low and dropping, and if calorie intake is low and dropping, then leptin levels drop. That signals the brain to turn appetite levels up and tells the thyroid to turn metabolic rate down.

When you're really lean, you're also at a higher risk of losing muscle. From a survival perspective, extra muscle is not beneficial when there's a calorie shortage. It's like having an engine that's bigger than you need. Muscle is a gas guzzler, and your body is trying to be more economical by downsizing the engine.

How to Break Any Fat-Loss Plateau

The best way to deal with plateaus is to avoid them in the first place. When you understand the physiology of calorie restriction, this may seem easier said than done. But you can put the odds in your favor by shunning extreme diets and losing weight at a slow and steady pace of about two pounds per week. When you resort to extreme methods, plateaus and weight regain are almost inevitable.

Even when you're sensible and conservative in your approach, at one time or another your weight loss may slow down and plateaus may occur. The good news is that it won't be a problem if you know the simple four-step process to break any plateau.

1. Check your compliance and raise your accountability. The first thing you should do if your weight loss has slowed or stopped is to double-check your compliance. How well did you follow your program over the last week? To ensure your compliance rate is on track for the next week, you should always journal your food intake when your progress has stopped. Use as many accountability tools as you can until you are back on track. Guesstimating your calories or eyeballing portions is fine if you're getting the results you want, but when you're stalled, it's time to get serious and start counting.

2. Reestablish your caloric deficit. If your nutrition and training compliance were spot-on, then you have to assume that you've started losing your caloric deficit due to metabolic adaptation or decreased calorie needs. The solution is simple: reestablish the caloric deficit. You have three choices about how you do this. One, you could increase your calorie expenditure by doing more cardio or doing your cardio with higher intensity. Two, you could decrease your caloric intake by cutting back on your food-portion sizes. Or three, you could do a little bit of both.

If you want to reduce your calories to break a plateau, that's where the X factor comes in. Instead of reducing all your calories across the board, selectively reduce the most calorie-dense carbohydrates. First, make sure there are no refined or processed sugars remaining in your diet. If there are, ditch them at once. Second, you can begin to selectively reduce starches and grains such as bread, pasta, and cereals. Once these lightly processed carbs have also been reduced, then you can even selectively reduce natural starches like potatoes, rice, and grains. Do not reduce your calories from protein, vegetables, or essential fats when reducing your caloric intake. A plateau-breaking diet is "lean, green, and marine"—lean protein, vegetables ("green"), and omega-3 fats such as salmon ("marine").

3. Go back to work with your adjusted strategy. After you've chosen the strategy of choice to reestablish your calorie deficit, go back to work for another seven days and measure your results again the following Monday. If it worked, keep it up. If it didn't work, repeat this process for as long as it's still practical (in other words, as long as you still have room to add more exercise or reduce calories without extremes). Otherwise, move on to the fourth strategy.

4. Take a diet break. If you're still struggling after going through the first three steps, then you might want to consider taking a diet break. This is the most counterintuitive of all the plateau-breaking strategies because a diet break means that you'll eat more by returning your calories to maintenance level for a full week. This is a strategy you should consider when you've been in a caloric deficit for at least three to four months.

Although you might expect to gain weight from doing this, it's usually only a few pounds and that's generally from increased glycogen storage. You won't gain fat if you only return your calories to maintenance. The increase in calories shuts off the starvation alarm, stimulates your metabolism, and resets the fat-burning and starvation hormones.

You also get a psychological break from the diet as well, which makes it easier to stick with the program when you go back to it. When you go back to your calorie deficit, your body will respond again the way it did when you first started the program.

Results-Based Thinking: The Secret to Continuous Progress

Fat loss is not a mystery. Progress plateaus are almost never caused by some unexplainable physiological anomaly. The simplest explanation is almost always the correct one: if your weight loss has stopped, you're no longer in a calorie deficit. The only real question to ask is, what happened to your calorie deficit?

Many people don't believe in the calories-in versus calories-out formula, and they say it's just a theory. This error is often made because they don't understand that energy balance is dynamic, which means that your calorie needs can change. A deficit for you today might not be a deficit for you six months from now.

Hopefully, you'll be a leaner person six months from now. If so, then you'll need fewer calories to maintain your lighter weight. Next to underestimating your calorie intake, forgetting to adjust your calorie intake when your energy needs change is the most common cause of plateaus and slow results.

It all boils down to one thing: results. Results-based thinking is the key to continuous progress and the solution to every body fat problem. Measure everything, get into a feedback loop, hold yourself accountable, and let your results dictate your approach.

Staying Lean and Staying Strong

Secrets of Maintaining Your Perfect Weight for Life

CHAPTER TWELVE

> ETERNAL vigilance is the price of freedom.
>
> —THOMAS JEFFERSON

Now that you're almost ready to get started, this seems like an appropriate time to make some predictions: follow the principles in this book and I predict that you will burn off fat and build lean muscle. You will master your emotions and develop a life-enriching relationship with food. You will develop a keen understanding of your mind and the effects your thoughts, beliefs, and attitudes have on your body and behavior. You *will* achieve your perfect weight goal.

267

That leads us to a crucial question: after you succeed, what then? How are you going to maintain your new body? What does your next set of twelve-week, six-month, and twelve-month goals look like? What's your next fitness challenge? What's going to keep you interested in training? How do you plan to stay motivated? What will prevent you from slipping back into old patterns?

There's a price you must pay to get what you want. There's also a price you must pay to keep it. You're not finished once you reach your ideal weight and body fat level. You're just beginning. It may seem like an oxymoron to approach maintenance with the attitude of continuous improvement, but if you do, it will be the start of an exciting and rewarding new lifestyle, not a tedious fight against backsliding.

Even better, your new lifestyle will eventually become automatic as long as you're willing to take a long-term perspective, develop new habits, and go through the full learning process rather than seek quick fixes. Your daily program will become so habitual you won't even have to think about it anymore. Eventually, your unconscious mind will run the whole show for you. Well, almost. You can never let down your guard or take your success for granted.

The Relapse Problem

A woman in a support group once said, "I'm an *expert* at losing weight because I lost two hundred pounds!" Everyone in the room gasped with respect and admiration. Then she finished her sentence. "Unfortunately, it was the same twenty pounds ten times." Relapse has always been a problem with health-related behavior change. Relapse rates for drug, alcohol, and tobacco dependency have been reported in the range of 50–90 percent. Relapse rates for weight loss are typically 70–90 percent, according to very reliable sources.

A study from Oxford University on weight maintenance and relapse published in *The International Journal of Obesity* confirmed the statistics we've all heard so often in the mass media:

IT'S A CONSISTENT FINDING that the weight lost by obese patients as a result of the most widely available treatments is almost always regained over time. Usually

about half the weight lost is regained in the first year with weight regain continuing thereafter, so that by three to five years posttreatment about 80 percent of patients have returned to, or even exceeded, their pretreatment weight.

Obviously, there are some big differences between substance-abuse relapse and weight relapse, namely the pharmacology of drugs, nicotine, and alcohol. But there are also some striking similarities, including the relapse statistics themselves. So similar are the mental and physical challenges that many people believe overeating and obesity are addictive disorders and should be treated as such.

Whether you think that regaining lost weight is as serious as substance-abuse relapse or not, don't take it lightly. Maintaining a stable lean body weight is a very important health goal. It's dangerous to repeatedly gain and lose weight. Research in animals and humans has revealed that weight cycling can make your metabolism less efficient.

After each bout of weight loss and regain, it becomes more difficult to burn fat the next time. You also become more predisposed to sudden weight regain if you binge or even if you reefed to previous maintenance levels. Long term, your body composition may get worse, as you lose large amounts of lean tissue during the weight-loss phase, but regain mostly fat on the rebound. In the end, you're heavier than when you started or you've become a skinny fat person.

Weight cycling has detrimental effects on your health as well. Usually, your blood pressure and blood cholesterol will go down in parallel with your body fat level. However, when you regain weight in repeated cycles, the negative effect on your blood pressure and cholesterol can be greater than the positive effects you got from losing the weight. Some experts even propose that weight cycling can shorten your life span.

Avoid These Weight Relapse Mistakes

One piece of good news is that the reasons for relapse are not a mystery. We know why weight regain happens and it's not difficult to predict. Weight relapsers have been studied in great depth and their behaviors are quite distinct from maintainers. You can avoid relapse right from the source of the problem if you take an inventory of which regainer behaviors you're engaging in and then avoid these mistakes in the future.

RELAPSE MISTAKE #1: Choosing the Wrong Diet to Lose the Weight

Maintenance begins with choosing the right nutrition program during the fat-loss phase. The first mistake that leads to relapse is following a diet so extreme or restrictive that it triggers bingeing or is simply too difficult to stay on for long. This includes not only the eating plan itself, but also any other weight-loss methods, such as supplements or drugs. One study published in the *American Journal of Clinical Nutrition* found that far more relapsers had lost weight by fasting or taking appetite suppressant pills than maintainers. Apparently, the fasting helped take some weight off and the pills helped curb hunger, but neither helped keep the weight off.

RELAPSE MISTAKE #2: Unrealistic Deadlines

Many authorities say that unrealistic weight goals are one of the biggest causes of failure and relapse. There's truth in that, but provided that body composition is kept in mind, I think the real problem is unrealistic deadlines, more so than unrealistic goals.

Most people sell themselves short and don't set their fitness standards high enough. Puny goals and low standards are set for one main reason: fear. By setting low standards, you don't risk disappointment. You can play it safe if you choose, but if you do, that's the same as accepting mediocrity. We all have genetic constraints and we can't change our inherent body structures, but as long as your goals aren't so outlandish that they're merely wishful thinking, I believe you should set big, ambitious goals. You simply have to be smart about choosing deadlines.

To calculate the time frame, divide your amount of weight loss desired by the ideal weekly weight-loss target of two pounds per week. If you want to drop thirty pounds, at two pounds per week, that's fifteen weeks. If you factor in some water-weight loss or above average fat loss, you might get there in twelve weeks. But if your goal is thirty pounds in thirty days, you'd better think twice about that deadline. Even if you met that deadline by dropping large amounts of water and lean tissue, it would have been counterproductive because there's a direct correlation between speed of weight loss and relapse.

RELAPSE MISTAKE #3: Abruptly Stopping a Nutrition or Exercise Program

Carmen was a forty-three-year-old mother of one whom I worked with several years ago. I remember her well because she experienced some of the best results I have ever seen. Her motivation was driven to an all-time high by entering a twelve-week before-and-after competition, which offered a hefty sum of prize money to the winner. She hired me to measure her body-fat percentage every week.

If you looked up "motivated' in the dictionary, you would see a picture of Carmen. She trained her butt off every day and got leaner every week, shedding a total of 10 percent body fat in twelve weeks without losing any lean body mass. At the end of the twelve weeks, she took her "after" photos in the best shape of her life. The last day I measured her body fat, her jeans were almost falling off her as she was literally jumping up and down for joy.

Then the strangest thing happened. As soon as the contest was over, she stopped training and dropped out of the gym overnight. My calls went unanswered for weeks. Months later, she finally turned up. She was heavier than before and very depressed about it. Carmen had not thought or planned a day beyond her twelve-week goal, so when the contest ended her reason to continue had ended.

She took for granted that the physique she developed from twelve weeks of serious effort could not be maintained without continued effort. You'd think this would be common sense, but research says otherwise. One study on long-term maintenance sponsored by the Kaiser Permanente HMO organization said that the relapsers seemed to assume that their lost weight was "permanently gone" and they were surprised when they found themselves heavy again.

RELAPSE MISTAKE #4: Returning to Your Previous Caloric Maintenance Level Without Increasing Activity

After a large weight loss, your calorie maintenance level is lower than it was when you started. With a fifty-pound weight loss, for example, an average guy will have a maintenance level about 400 calories lower than when he started his fat-loss phase. Do you see the conundrum? If he goes back to his old maintenance level, and all else remains equal, he is *guaranteed* to regain the weight. The math equation has changed.

Even if you're aware of this potential pitfall, permanently reducing your calories to accommodate your new energy requirements is one of those "easier said than done" propositions. If you've gotten accustomed to eating a certain volume of food for years or even for an entire lifetime, it's not always an easy adjustment to make. You have two choices. One, you can get used to eating less than you did before your weight loss. Two, you can get used to exercising more. Ideally, you'll do a little bit of both and that will make life easiest.

This reduction in calorie needs after weight loss explains why increasing exercise has always been the single most cited success strategy for long-term weight maintenance. The increased activity offsets the lower maintenance level and it's easier for most people to stay active than it is for them to eat less than they were previously used to.

RELAPSE MISTAKE #5: Dichotomous Thinking

Relapsers see situations in black-and-white terms without shades of gray. For example, they insist they have no time to train rather than making efficient use of what little time they have. They're either on the program completely or off completely. If they have one bad meal, they feel as if their entire week has been completely ruined. If they miss a deadline, instead of just pushing back the date, they think they blew an entire twelve weeks.

Relapsers also have very rigid ideas of what success means. For example, they might define success as weighing 125 pounds and anything other than 125 pounds is seen as a failure. Fitness is not a win-or-lose, pass-or-fail situation. Fitness is a journey of learning and self-improvement. All-or-none thinking creates unnecessary stress and doesn't allow you to give yourself credit for what you did right or to learn from your experiences. Cut yourself some slack and avoid this mistake in thinking at all costs.

RELAPSE MISTAKE #6: Perpetual Dissatisfaction with Body Weight and Shape

Relapsers express great dissatisfaction with their new body weight and body shape, even when they've made huge strides in progress. They tend to make comparisons of themselves to others and when taken to an extreme, this turns into perfectionism where no achievement ever seems good enough. Relapsers also tend to make judgments about themselves as people strictly on the basis of their physical attributes.

The pursuit of constant improvement is clearly a virtue. Some of the healthiest and fittest people in the world credit their success to never becoming complacent and always striving for better results. This seems to be in conflict with body dissatisfaction as a cause of relapse. We can reconcile this paradox by understanding that you can strive for continuous improvement while also liking yourself at every step along the way—it's not one or the other.

It's also important to get very clear about how far you want to take your physical development and how much time and effort you're willing to invest. Not everyone wants or needs the washboard abs of a *Men's Health* cover model or the body shape of a figure model. Use 80-20 thinking here. Suppose you can get 80 percent of the way to what you consider your physical ideal with a fairly modest investment of time and effort. To capture the next 15 percent takes more time and serious hard work, and the final 5 percent takes a monumental full-time effort. How far to you want to go and how much are you willing to pay?

RELAPSE MISTAKE #7: Poor Coping and Stress Management Skills

High levels of stress, unexpected life events, and negative emotions can all lead to weight regain if you don't have strong coping mechanisms to deal with them. Maintainers experience the same nonhealth stresses that relapsers do: financial difficulties, family issues, and work stress. The difference is, relapsers use food to distract themselves or escape from bad feelings rather than confront their problems head-on and develop alternate coping mechanisms.

Women need to be more on guard than men. According to the Styles survey, which was conducted to identify characteristics of weight maintainers, more men (35.5 percent) were successful at maintenance than women (27.7 percent). The most likely reason for this difference is that women are sometimes more emotional than men and may be more susceptible to emotional eating.

Regardless of your gender, to maintain your weight, you have to continue reminding yourself that food is for fuel, for nourishment, and for bodybuilding material, not for coping with stress. If you haven't mastered stress management and developed good coping skills during the fat-loss phase, then it will be a struggle to maintain your weight goal even if you manage to reach it.

Listen to Maintainers, Not to Losers

Today, it's the media and advertising-hyped stories of rapid weight loss and dramatic before-and-after transformations that get all the attention. It's easy to look at these "success stories" and choose them as your role models. But it's not the person who lost the most weight or who lost weight the fastest that you want to emulate. Large weight loss could mean that a lot of muscle tissue or water weight was lost. Rapid weight loss prompts the question of how long that weight loss has been and will be maintained.

When you're looking for people and methods to model, you should pay attention to maintainers, not losers. Maintainers are people who have held a steady ideal weight for one year or longer. Long-term maintainers are people who have kept the weight off for three to five years. Anytime you meet or hear about people who have achieved their ideal weight and maintained it for more than five years, stop everything you're doing, pay attention, and learn from them.

Finding long-term maintainers is not easy. First of all, and sadly, there aren't that many yet. Second, most commercial diet programs don't keep track of their customers over the long term. The testimonials they publish are the most dramatic success stories that have been singled out as their poster children. From a business point of view, you can't fault them for that, but the results you see in the ads are almost never a true reflection of the usual amount of weight loss or the duration of weight-loss maintenance. That's why the FTC requires disclaimers such as "results not typical" on the bottom of so many advertisements and before-and-after photos.

One group dedicated to tracking the maintainers is the National Weight Control Registry (NWCR). This joint collaboration of weight-loss researchers was founded in 1994 by Dr. James Hill, a clinical nutrition researcher from the University of Colorado, and Dr. Rena Wing, a psychologist from Brown University.

The NWCR began as a database of men and women who had lost thirty pounds or more and maintained the loss for one year or more. Since its inception, the average participant has been even more successful than the entry criteria, having lost an average of sixty-five pounds and maintained the minimum weight loss for an average period of five and a half years.

Information about this group has been collected through a series of surveys and interviews. Since this isn't the controlled experimental type of research, it doesn't prove cause and effect and is subject to flaws such as selection bias and the ever-present underreporting bias. Nevertheless, the NWCR is one of the most valuable sources of success strategies from weight maintainers currently available. Many of the strategies in the ten major keys to maintenance are based on the findings of this group and other groups like them.

The Ten Major Keys for Successful Lifelong Maintenance

The NWCR found many similarities among successful maintainers plus a few important differences. One difference was the type of program used. Half of the maintainers lost weight on their own, while half of them used commercial programs. Maintainers also used various types of nutrition programs with a variety of different macronutrient ratios, and they customized their nutrition programs to suit their needs, lifetyles, and dispositions.

This shows that it wasn't a specific formal program that made the difference. It tells us that personal preference and metabolic individuality must be taken into consideration when choosing a program. No one can say that a single program is superior to all the others 100 percent of the time for 100 percent of people.

Despite the differences, the NWCR and similar survey studies reveal that maintainers have far more in common than they have different. It's these commonalities in long-term maintainers you'll want to learn and emulate.

1. Maintainers Have a Plan for Transitioning into Maintenance Phase

The worst thing you can do at the time you reach your weight goal is to abruptly end a diet and make sudden changes to totally different foods or a dramatically different quantity of food. The stricter your diet has been, the more important it is to include a gradual transition plan to take you from your caloric deficit level to your new maintenance level. If your calorie reduction and food restrictions were very conservative, you won't need much of a transition period; you should be able to safely bring your calories right up to maintenance without a problem.

A transition phase might take place over the course of one week, or it might stretch out as long as three to four weeks if your diet was very restrictive and you are prone to sudden weight gain. Your objective is to slowly establish energy balance so your weight stabilizes. As you bring your calories back up to maintenance, use the weekly feedback method and continue to monitor your weight and body composition.

Remember that body weight is not the same as body fat, so don't be alarmed if there is a small weight gain, provided your body-fat percentage does not increase significantly. Sometimes you'll gain two to three pounds, but it's usually lean tissue, water, and muscle glycogen, especially if you had reduced your carbs during the fat-loss phase. When your weight is stable and you're neither gaining nor losing week to week, you know you're in energy balance and you've officially entered the maintenance phase, or if you prefer, the "lifestyle phase."

2. Maintainers Have Very High Levels of Physical Activity

One thing that almost every weight-loss expert agrees on is that exercise and high levels of activity are the number one key to keeping off the weight. That's not to say it's impossible to keep weight off with no activity, only that it's difficult. It would take very tight control over caloric intake and high levels of dietary restraint to maintain a large weight loss with no training or other physical activity during the maintenance phase.

The reason that maintenance is difficult without exercise is that after a large loss of body weight your caloric needs are lower than they were before. It's a bad idea to abruptly end your diet the minute you reach your weight goal and go back to the way you used to eat. It's an even worse idea to abruptly stop exercising.

There have been many studies investigating the ideal amount of exercise for weight maintenance, and while the experts agree that exercise is important for maintenance, they can't seem to agree on how much. You may have heard news stories claiming everything from "thirty minutes of moderate physical activity most days of the week" to "an hour a day or more." It's hard to make heads or tails out of it all.

My suggestion is to simply continue following the Body Fat Solution training guidelines. Perform three days per week of strength training, three days a week of formal, moderate to intense cardio training, and keep up an active lifestyle in general. If you were doing more than three days per week of cardio, you will probably be able to reduce back to the baseline level of three days per week.

Adjust your activity level as needed based on your results just like you did during the fat-loss phase. Why be bound by rigid rules or confusing research? A simple weigh-in and body fat test will tell you without a shred of doubt.

3. Maintainers Decrease Sedentary Activities

Long-term maintainers are much more active than regainers, but they also make a conscious effort to cut back on sedentary recreational activities. It's not just what you do that counts, it's what you don't do. When you stop doing something sedentary, that will create a vacuum that begs to be filled, so to make the change stick, swap out the time you used to spend watching TV, surfing the Web, playing video games, or just lounging around for some kind of physical activity.

The best part of this strategy is that the new activity could still be recreational and fun, it simply has to burn some calories. Think about all the possibilities. This could be a great opportunity to take up some new sports or hobbies like surfing, boating, Jet Skiing, hiking, gardening, golf, bowling, or tennis. These may not take the place of your formal cardio program, and definitely can't take the place of weight training, but they will make a difference in helping you stay lean if you make them a part of your new lifestyle.

If you're not a gym person, using this strategy can also help reduce the amount of time you need to spend on formal training. If you're serious about maintenance, you're going to need to stay active. But there's no law that says you have to be indoors on a treadmill seven days a week, unless you want to.

4. Maintainers Get Serious About Weight Training

The types of exercise regimes used by maintainers may vary, but in the majority of studies, maintainers reported that they used weight training to help take the weight off and continued weight training through the maintenance phase. The majority of regainers didn't do weight training during the weight loss phase, and most didn't pick it up in the maintenance phase.

Years ago, I did my own informal research on weight training and maintenance by looking at the habits and long-term results of several hundred of my personal training and coaching program graduates. They all used weight training as a part of their fat-loss programs. Of course, my sample was biased because lifting weights was mandatory. But I noticed something else. Afterward, the most successful of my clients were the ones who got extremely serious about their weight training to the point that it almost became like a hobby or recreational sport to them. A few even took up bodybuilding or figure competitions.

I believe the progressive and goal-oriented nature of weight training adds a motivational spark that keeps the fire of enthusiasm burning for years after you achieve your initial weight goal. Contrary to what many believe about exercise and aging, weight training is also a sport you can enjoy for the rest of your life. There's no other type of exercise that will do so much for you as you get older to maintain your strength, functionality, mobility, confidence, and self-esteem.

5. Maintainers Continue Diligent Self-monitoring

Research has proven over and over again that people who monitor their progress have a higher chance of succeeding at reaching their body fat goals. What clinches the deal is that self-monitoring of body weight and other measures of progress increase your chances for successful maintenance as well.

Among maintainers, the five most common self-monitoring methods include:

- tracking body weight;
- tracking calories;
- planning meals;
- tracking dietary fat intake;
- measuring the amount of food.

Among the NWCR maintainers who lost sixty-five pounds or more and kept if off for at least five years, 75 percent of them reported weighing themselves at least once a week. Many weighed themselves daily. Once you hit your target weight, don't put that scale away just yet. Weighing yourself not only helps you take the weight off, it helps you keep it off.

6. Maintainers Respond Quickly to Counteract Weight Gain

One of the reasons that self-monitoring behaviors help so much is that they give you an early warning system to help put a lid on the weight creep. Putting a stop to creeping body weight also requires a certain mind-set. The first part is a low level of tolerance for weight gain. Most successful maintainers have set a rule for how much weight they'll allow themselves to gain before they spring into corrective action.

Four pounds is a commonly cited figure. This makes perfect sense because most people say their normal weight fluctuation is about two to three pounds. As soon as they exceed that limit, they leap into action. When the early warning alarm goes off, they immediately go back into a caloric deficit by reducing food portions or increasing the number of calories burned through formal exercise.

The other side of killing the weight creep monster while it's small is having high standards for the type of physique you want to maintain or develop. In my opinion, many trainers and nutrition professionals wimp out when it comes to helping people set their long-term fitness goals. Their intentions are good, as they don't want their clients to be unrealistic, but I think it would do a lot more good if they encouraged their clients to raise their standards.

The majority of maintainers I know believe that it's not okay to be overweight and it's dangerous to be obese. Other people, usually those who are struggling with their weight, argue that you have to accept yourself the way you are to be a mentally healthy, happy, well-adjusted human being. I don't think anyone would disagree with that, except that this is dichotomous thinking. Fat and a person are separate things, so you don't have to accept them together. Fat is not a person, it's a temporary physical condition. The person you are is much more than a mass of biological tissue. You can like and accept yourself as a person and at the same time proclaim that high body fat is unacceptable.

Unrealistic standards are certainly a possibility, so set yours based on what you really want, not what society says or implies is the ideal. Raising standards doesn't mean getting skinnier and skinnier. High standards include excellent body composition and all the other aspects of fitness, including strength, muscularity, endurance, flexibility, and aerobic capacity. But almost all of us are so far away from our true physical potential and have so much room for improvement that it's silly to downsize our goals and dreams because someone else thinks they're unrealistic.

7. Maintainers Follow the Seven Lifestyle Eating Habits

The eating habits that help to keep the weight off are almost identical to the nutrition habits that take the fat off. However, in virtually all of the long-term studies about weight maintenance, seven lifestyle eating habits in particular show up at the top of the list over and over again.

Successful maintainers:

- Eat at least five fruits and vegetables per day. You can never hear this often enough: Eat more fruits and vegetables. They're great for burning the fat off, great for keeping the fat off.
- Eat a high-fiber diet. Successful maintainers report a high-fiber intake from their high fruit and vegetable intake, as well as from other natural starchy carb and whole-grain sources, such as beans, oats, legumes, brown rice, sweet potatoes, and barley.
- Eat breakfast every day. It's no surprise that maintainers are breakfast eaters because strong correlations have been found between skipping breakfast and overeating or bingeing later in the day.
- Eat at fast-food restaurants no more than two times per week. A report on dietary practices and dining-out behavior published by the Centers for Disease Control found that adults who ate no more than two times per week at fast-food restaurants were more successful at maintenance.
- Eat less dietary fat. Most maintainers report eating between 20 percent and 30 percent of their total calories from fat, significantly less than the national average of 35 percent. It's important to consume enough of the healthy fats, but maintainers are aware that high-fat foods are high-calorie foods, so quantities are controlled.

- Eat consciously. Long-term maintainers are not mindless eaters. Even though healthy eating behaviors become habitual after years of repetition, successful maintainers are always vigilant and aware.

- Eat the same healthy foods all year round. Maintainers eat a wide variety of foods, but they are consistent all year round. There's no dramatic difference between the foods eaten for maintenance because no weird or different foods are eaten for fat loss. To hold their weight steady, maintainers simply eat a little less of the same healthy foods during the fat-loss phrase.

8. Maintainers Continue Using Social Support

I remember the first time I ever heard about lifetime memberships for weight-loss programs. My first reaction was, "What a rip-off. Why would you need a lifetime membership if the program actually worked?" After I started doing research and I discovered that ongoing social support was one of the secrets of successful maintenance, I realized that these programs weren't just a money grab. Of course, if you've been offered a purchase plan for fat-burning pills with lifetime refills and monthly autoshipping, you might want to think twice about that one. I'm talking about professional coaching or support.

Not only do maintainers seek support from professionals, but they also use their natural social network to help them cope with personal problems. Regainers, on the other hand, lack coping skills, try to handle problems alone, and lapse back into using food as a coping mechanism.

If you choose to continue with coaching, counseling, or membership in some kind of fitness group, you can rest assured it will be one of the best investments you ever make. I take my own advice, by the way. I always realized that even the best athletes in the world have coaches and trainers, so why not me? I've been with the same personal trainer for twelve years. When I'm not working with him, I usually work out with a training partner.

Whether you work with a professional into the maintenance phase is your decision, but if you've ever relapsed in the past, give serious consideration to using professional support for a specified period after you reach your ideal weight. Most of the people who get past the one-year mark have good prospects for maintaining their new weight for the long term, so having a coach or trainer for that period would be a great idea. Even if you don't keep your trainer for years, like I have, yours can at least help you make the smoothest possible transition into maintenance.

9. Maintainers Become Coaches and Role Models

Support is a circle, not a one-way transaction. Someone gives support, someone receives it, and then the receiving party either returns the favor to the same person or "pays it forward" to someone else. One of the best maintenance strategies is becoming a coach and support partner after you achieve your goals. Not only will you be returning the goodwill you received from others when you needed help, you'll be keeping yourself motivated by taking a leadership position where others are looking up to you. To avoid disappointing them, you have to be congruent and practice what you preach.

Being a coach or support friend for others could be as simple as posting your success story on a website or contributing to an online community. You might even become involved in the health and fitness business more formally. I believe that part of our purpose on this earth is to serve other people. When you serve others, you get an incredible feeling you can't get any other way. Emotional eaters use food as a way to make themselves feel better, but food wasn't meant for that purpose. Try service if you want a way to genuinely feel better.

Give something back. Do it for selfish reasons if no other, because being a role model for others helps you achieve your own goals. Imagine what would happen if every person who achieved and maintained their ideal weight "paid it forward" by helping three other people reach and maintain their ideal weight. Maybe that's just a cute idea from a movie. But maybe it's much more.

10. Maintainers Have Vision

Some people may wonder why the Body Fat Solution isn't a seven-day makeover, a six-week program, or a twelve-week transformation contest. As you may have noticed, I do recommend setting short, mid- and long-term goals, including twelve-week goals. I recommend planning by the seven-day week, and I suggest setting up your training in neatly organized four-week blocks and eight-week cycles. I also think competitions are a great idea.

But the answer is that the Body Fat Solution is a lifestyle, not a twelve-week program. Forgive me the cliché, but there's no better approach to nutrition, training, and health than thinking of fitness as a lifestyle. Programs and goals are just stepping-stones, not the journey itself.

If the only plans you make are for winning a twelve-week transformation contest or for looking good for a trip to the beach in thirty days, what's going to keep you going after that? Even five-, ten-, and twenty-year goals have an ending point. What then? That's where a vision comes into play. A vision is the big picture of what you want for your body and your health, but unlike a goal, a vision has no end point. You don't arrive there or get it, you live it.

Putting a man on the moon before the end of the decade was a goal. The exploration and conquest of space is a vision. If there was no vision, would anyone be talking about going to Mars today?

Here are a few more examples:

Goal: To win the Ms. Fitness America championship.
Vision: To become the best natural fitness competitor I can be.

Goal: To lose a hundred pounds.
Vision: To easily maintain my ideal weight, improve my health, increase my quality of life, and inspire other people with my success story.

Goal: To complete a full triathlon.
Vision: To continuously improve my performance and become the best athlete I can be.

Goal: To own a health club.

Vision: To build a national fitness company that inspires thousands of people to achieve their health and fitness goals.

Each time you achieve a goal, you have to keep asking, what's next? But if you have no vision, you'll be at a loss for an answer. If you have a vision, the next step is an obvious and natural progression. What's your big picture? What's your vision? Think about it hard and write it down. Then think about it some more and make it clearer and clearer. Vision, the never-ending pursuit of new goals, and personal improvement will be the driving forces that inspire, motivate, and energize you for the rest of your life.

The Final Step Is . . . Take the First Step

You now have all the tools you need to burn fat, build lean muscle, and maintain your perfect weight for life. What's the difference between this time and all the others when you didn't get results, when you relapsed, or you lacked the motivation to even get started? The difference is, you now see the full picture. Before, you only had isolated pieces. You now know that to solve a body fat problem, you have to attack it from the root causes in every area of your life—physical, mental, emotional, and social—and you now have a step-by-step success plan to do it.

With this knowledge at your fingertips, you should be feeling pretty excited and optimistic. But it's also natural to feel a bit intimidated by a new endeavor like this. After all, this book has covered a lot of ground, and we're talking about an entire change of lifestyle and mind-set, not just a diet. As you get ready to begin, remember two important points:

First, you can tackle your new lifestyle changes one at a time, if that's your choice. Some people are going to dive into this program headfirst and use every strategy in the book right from the beginning. But if that's not your style, choose the one part of your lifestyle that needs the most work, and start working on that today. Set one small goal for this week, take action, and achieve it. Plan. Prioritize. Take the first step. That's how you get anywhere and that's how you take the overwhelm out of anything.

Second, most of the changes you'll work hard to make initially are eventually going to become almost effortless. You always have to stay on top of your game, just as a virtuoso musician or world-class athlete must always practice to avoid losing his skill. However, your unconscious mind, if trained and programmed with enough repetition and emotional intensity, has the capacity to almost completely take over every behavior necessary for the long-term maintenance of your ideal body weight.

A healthy and well-trained body will automatically regulate your physiology. A healthy and well-trained mind will automatically regulate your behavior. And that's exactly what's going to happen if you train your mind and your body at the same time: this will all become automatic. It will become your new lifestyle. Achieving your goals is going to take hard work and it's going to take self-discipline and vigilance to keep what you've earned. But the longer you travel this path, the easier it gets, and I promise you, the rewards are worth it.

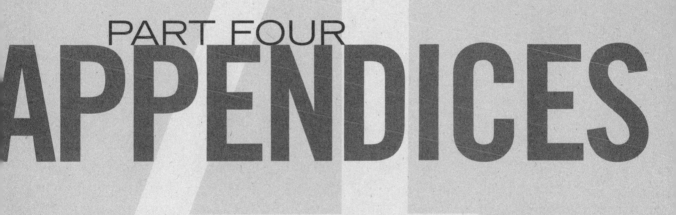

PART FOUR

APPENDICES

Appendix 1

Stay **Connected,** Get **Support,** and **Learn More** at The Body Fat Solution **Online**

- Sign up for our free e-mail newsletter so you can stay connected and get live updates as they're released.
- Get information about the Body Fat Solution online discussion groups and our inner circle support community.
- Connect with like-minded people, make new friends, and find accountability partners.
- Find Body Fat Solution–friendly recipes, menu plans, and cooking tips.
- Learn new exercises, discover new training techniques, and take your workouts to the next level.

www.TheBodyFatSolution.com

Appendix 2
Calorie Calculations

The ten Body Fat Solution nutrition rules are designed to help keep you away from number crunching as much as possible. By putting yourself into a feedback loop and using results-based thinking, calculating or counting calories becomes optional.

All you have to do is acknowledge the energy balance equation, become aware of your portion sizes, and then increase or decrease your portions based on your weekly results.

That said, the importance of maintaining a calorie deficit to burn fat can't be emphasized enough. If you're going to track numbers, calories are the most important number to know.

There are four methods to calculate your caloric needs. Depending on whether you're the analytical type or the "ballpark figure" type, select the method that suits your style the best.

1. The averages method

Use this method if you want a general ballpark figure and you don't like math!

For fat loss:

Men: 2100–2500 calories/day
Women: 1400–1800 calories/day

For maintenance:

Men: 2700–2900 calories/day
Women: 2000–2100 calories/day

2. The quick method

Use this formula if you want a personalized ballpark figure with one quick calculation. Use the lower number for lightly active, the middle number for moderately active, and the higher number for very active.

For fat loss:

10–12 calories per lb of body weight

For maintenance:

14–16 calories per lb of body weight

3. Harris-Benedict formula

Use this formula for a very accurate estimate of your maintenance level if you know your body weight but not your body fat percentage. For fat loss, create a 20–30 percent deficit below maintenance.

Note: BMR = basal metabolic rate, which is the amount of energy you require for normal body functions at rest (does not include activity).

Men: BMR = 66 + (13.7 × wt in kg) + (5 × ht in cm) = (6.8 × age in years)
Women: BMR = 655 + (9.6 × wt in kg) + (1.8 × ht in cm) = (4.7 × age in years)
Note: 1 inch = 2.54 cm
1 kilogram = 2.2 lbs

Example:

You are female
You are 30 years old
You are 5'6" tall (167.6 cm)
You weigh 120 lbs (54.5 kg)
Your BMR = 655 + 523 + 302 = 141 = 1339 calories/day

Now that you know your BMR, you can calculate your maintenance level, (also known as total daily energy expenditure or TDEE), by multiplying your BMR by your activity multiplier from the chart below:

Activity Multiplier:

Sedentary = BMR × 1.2 (little or no exercise, desk job)
Lightly active = BMR × 1.375 (light exercise/sports 1–3 days/week)
Moderately active = BMR × 1.55 (moderate exercise/sports 3–5 days/week)
Very active = BMR × 1.725 (hard exercise/sports 6–7 days/week)
Extremely active = BMR × 1.9 (hard daily exercise/sports and physical job or 2X day training, i.e., marathon, competition, etc.)

Example:

Your BMR is 1339 calories/day

Your activity level is moderately active (work out 3–5 times per week)

Your activity factor is 1.55

Your TDEE = 1.55 × 1339 = 2075 calories/day

4. Katch-McArdle formula

Use this formula for a very accurate estimate of your maintenance level if you know your body fat percentage and lean body mass. For fat loss, create a 20–30 percent deficit below maintenance.

BMR (men and women) = 370 + (21.6 × lean mass in kg)

Example:

You are female

You weigh 120 lbs (54.5 kg)

Your body fat percentage is 20% (24 lbs fat, 96 lbs lean)

Your lean mass is 96 lbs (43.6 kg)

Your BMR = 370 + (21.6 × 43.6) = 1312 calories/day

To determine TDEE from BMR, you simply multiply BMR by the activity
    multiplier:

Your BMR is 1312 calories/day

Your activity level is moderately active (working out 3–5 times per week)

Your activity factor is 1.55

Your TDEE = 1.55 × 1312 = 2033 calories/day

Appendix 3

Body Fat Solution
Recommended Foods

There are several ways you can use the Body Fat Solution recommended foods list:

1. To help you choose the best foods.

These lists provide you with all the best foods for getting a leaner and healthier body. This is not a comprehensive database of all prepared foods or list of foods to avoid. You won't see restaurant foods, fast food, or anything highly processed on these lists. There are many fine calorie-counter books and websites you can refer to if you ever want that information. Many people already have a good idea of what they shouldn't eat. Refer to these lists anytime you want to know what you should eat.

2. To give you ideas for variety.

If you ever get bored eating the same thing every day, these lists will stimulate you with fresh new ideas. Tired of apples and bananas? Try something more exotic like mangoes or papayas. Sick of chicken? How about buffalo, pork tenderloin, or even venison for lean protein? Bored with oatmeal every morning?

Why not sample a multigrain hot cereal with barley, triticale, rye, oats, and flax, and top it with fresh raspberries?

3. To create menus.

If you choose to count your calories or to create menus by the numbers (protein, carbs, and fats), these databases will help you do it. There are websites and software applications that can assist with the menu-planning process, but creating menus can be as simple as using these food lists to put together well-balanced meals. Simply choose a lean protein, add one or two natural sources of carbs, allow a small amount of healthy fat, and you have yourself a meal. Adjust the calories and portion sizes to suit your needs.

4. To raise your calorie awareness.

Even if you decide not to count calories, simply being more aware of calorie counts in general will influence your decisions in a big way. Did you ever munch on a full cup of raisins as a snack without realizing it contained 500 calories? How about peanut butter? Did you know three tablespoons sets you back almost 300 calories? Some foods are nutrient-dense, healthy, and make the recommended list, but they have a very high calorie density, so portion sizes must be strictly controlled.

About Serving Sizes and Recipes

For your convenience, all foods are listed with a serving size in volume, weight in ounces, and weight in grams. Keep in mind that the uncooked weights and cooked weights will vary and that will affect the calorie amounts. Meats lose fluids during cooking, so four ounces cooked will have more calories than four ounces raw (less fluid equals higher calorie density). Rice and pasta absorb water and expand during cooking, so they will contain more calories per unit of volume dry than cooked.

The majority of the foods listed are individual (one-ingredient) food items. Once you learn which individual foods are best to eat, then it's easy to combine them into your favorite healthy recipes. Any type of herbs and spices may be used to flavor your foods, and many herbs have healthful properties that make them superfoods in their own right. For recipe and menu ideas, be sure to visit the Body Fat Solution website at www.TheBodyFatSolution.com.

Body Fat Solution Recommended Foods

Lean Proteins

Food Item	Qty/wt	Weight/grams	Calories	Protein	Carbs	Fat	Fiber
Beef, flank steak, lean	4 oz uncooked	113	256	30	0	14.2	0.0
Beef, ground, 90% lean	4 oz uncooked	113	199	22.7	0	11.3	0.0
Beef, ground 95% lean	4 oz uncooked	113	155	24.3	0	6.0	0.0
Beef, round, eye of, lean	4 oz uncooked	113	198	32.9	0	6.5	0.0
Beef, round tip, lean	4 oz uncooked	113	213	32.6	0	8.3	0.0
Beef round, top, lean	4 oz uncooked	113	214	35.9	0	6.7	0.0
Beef, sirloin, top, lean	4 oz uncooked	113	229	34.4	0	9.1	0.0
Beef, tenderloin (filet)	4 oz uncooked	113	252	32	0	12.7	0.0
Buffalo (bison) steak, top round	4 oz uncooked	113	195	32.0	0	6.8	0.0
Chicken, canned	4 oz	113	100	18	0	2.0	0.0
Chicken breast, ground, lean	4 oz uncooked	113	100	24	0	0.5	0.0
Chicken breast, light meat, skinless	4 oz uncooked	113	196	35.1	0	5.1	0.0
Clams, raw	1/2 cup (4 oz)	113	84	14.5	2.9	1.1	0.0
Crab, fresh, raw (Dungeness, U.S. King, or stone)	4 oz	113	95	20.8	0	0.7	0.0
Crawfish	4 oz raw meat only	113	87	18.1	0	1.1	0.0
Egg whites, large	6	198	102	21	1.8	0.0	0.0
Egg whites, liquid	1 cup (8.6 oz)	244	120	26	1	0.0	0.0
Egg, whole, large	1	50	75	6.3	0.6	5.0	0.0

Food Item	Qty/wt	Weight/grams	Calories	Protein	Carbs	Fat	Fiber
Elk (game meat)	4 oz roasted	113	166	34.2	0	2.2	0.0
Fish, bass, striped	4 oz raw	113	110	20.1	0	2.7	0.0
Fish, catfish	4 oz raw	113	108	18.6	0	3.3	0.0
Fish, cod, Pacific	4 oz uncooked	113	93	20.2	0	0.8	0.0
Fish, flounder (flatfish)	4 oz uncooked	113	104	21.4	0	1.4	0.0
Fish, halibut, Pacific	4 oz uncooked	113	124	23.6	0	2.6	0.0
Fish, mackerel, Atlantic	4 oz uncooked	113	230	21	0	15.8	0.0
Fish, mackerel, canned in olive oil	1 can (3.9 oz)	110 g	290	24	0	22.0	0.0
Fish, mackerel, Pacific (jack)	4 oz uncooked	113	179	22.8	0	9.0	0.0
Fish, pollack	4 oz uncooked	113	104	22.1	0	1.1	0.0
Fish, rainbow trout	4 oz uncooked	113	135	23.2	0	3.9	0.0
Fish, salmon (wild)	4 oz	113	206	28.8	0	9.2	0.0
Fish, tilapia	4 oz uncooked	113	110	23	0	2.0	0.0
Fish, tuna, canned in water, albacore	4 oz	113	140	26	0	2.0	0.0
Fish, tuna, canned in water, chunk light	4 oz	113	120	26	0	1.0	0.0
Fish, tuna, yellowfin (tuna steak)	4 oz uncooked	113	123	26.5	0	1.1	0.0
Lamb, loin	4 oz roasted	113	217	32.1	0	8.8	0.0
Lobster	4 oz uncooked	113	102	21.3	0.6	1.0	0.0
Mahi-mahi, U.S.	4 oz raw	113	97	21	0	0.8	0.0
Mussels	4 oz raw	113	98	13.5	4.2	2.5	0.0
Ostrich steak	4 oz uncooked	113	135	28	0	3.5	0.0
Oysters, Pacific	4 oz raw	113	92	10.7	5.6	2.6	0.0
Pork tenderloin	4 oz uncooked	113	136	23.8	0	3.9	0.0
Prawns	4 oz raw	113	119	22.7	1	1.9	0.0
Protein powder, casein (a milk protein)	1 scoop	31	110	23	3	0.5	1.0
Protein powder, hemp (vegetarian)	1 scoop	31	110	23	3	0.5	1.0
Protein powder, soy (vegetarian)	1 scoop	31	120	25	2	1.5	0.0
Protein powder, whey (a milk protein)	1 scoop	24	90	18	2	2.0	0.0
Salmon burgers	1 burger (3.2 oz)	91	80	18	1	0.1	1.0
Salmon, canned, pink	4 oz	113	90	0	5	0.0	0.0
Salmon, wild Alaskan	4 oz	113	206	28.8	0	9.2	0.0
Sardines (herring), canned in olive oil	1 can (3.2 oz)	91	191	22.7	0	10.5	0.0

Food Item	Qty.	Weight/grams	Calories	Protein	Carbs	Fat	Fiber
Sardines (herring), canned in water	1 can (3.2 oz)	91	150	19	0	8.0	0.0
Scallops	4 oz raw	113	100	19	2.7	0.9	0.0
Shrimp	4 oz	113	120	23	1	2.0	0.0
Squid	4 oz raw	113	104	17.7	3.5	1.6	0.0
Tempeh (vegetarian protein)	1/2 cup (2.9 oz)	82	160	15.4	7.8	9.0	3.3
Tofu, firm, raw (vegetarian protein)	2.9 oz	117	117	12.8	3.5	7.1	0.0
Turkey breast, skinless	4 oz	113	178	33.9	0	3.7	0.0
Turkey, ground 99% lean	4 oz	113	120	28	0	1.0	0.0
Venison steak	4 oz	113	173	35	0	2.3	0.0

Starchy Vegetables, Grains, Beans & Legumes (Natural Complex Carbs) X2

Food Item	Qty.	Weight/grams	Calories	Protein	Carbs	Fat	Fiber
Beans, adzuki, canned	1/2 cup (4.1 oz)	116	147	8.7	28.5	0.1	8.4
Beans, black, canned	1/2 cup (4.6 oz)	130	100	7	20	0.5	8
Beans, garbanzo (chickpeas), canned	1/2 cup (4.6 oz)	130	120	7	19	1.5	5
Beans, kidney, canned	1/2 cup (4.5 oz)	127	110	7	20	0.5	8
Beans, navy, canned	1/2 cup (4.6 oz)	130	110	7	20	0.5	7
Beans, pinto, canned	1/2 cup (4.2 oz)	119	100	6	18	0	6
Black-eyed peas, canned or frozen	1/2 cup (4.6 oz)	130	90	6	16	1	4
Cassava (yuca root)	1/2 cup (3.5 oz)	99	165	1.4	39.2	0.3	1.8
Chickpeas (garbanzos), canned	1/2 cup (4.6 oz)	130	120	7	19	1.5	5
Corn, canned	1/2 cup (5.4 oz)	153	70	2	18	1	3
Lentils	1/2 cup cooked (3.5 oz)	99	115	9	20	0	7.8
Lima beans, canned	1/2 cup (4.5 oz)	127	120	7	23	1	8
Oatmeal, old-fashioned (no sugar added)	1/2 cup dry (1.4 oz)	40	150	5	27	3	4
Oatmeal, steel-cut (no sugar added)	1/4 cup dry (1.4 oz)	40	150	5	27	2.5	4
Plantains	1/2 med (3.9 oz)	110	180	0	22	0	5
Potato, sweet	1 med uncooked (6 oz)	170	136	2.1	31.6	0.4	3.9
Potato, white	1 lg uncooked (7 oz)	198	160	4.2	36.3	0.2	3.2
Rice, brown, basmati, cooked	1 cup (8.6 oz)	6.9	216	5	44.8	1.8	3.6
Rice, brown, basmati, dry	1/2 cup dry (3.3 oz)	94	320	8	64	3	4
Rice, brown, long-grain, cooked	1 cup cooked (6.8 oz)	96	216	5	44.8	1.8	3.6
Rice, brown, long-grain, dry	1/2 cup dry (3.3 oz)	94	320	8	64	3	4
Rice, wild, cooked	1 cup (5.8 oz)	164	166	6.5	35	0.6	1.5

Starchy Vegetables, Grains, Beans & Legumes (Natural Complex Carbs) X2 *(cont.)*

Food Item	Qty.	Weight/grams	Calories	Protein	Carbs	Fat	Fiber
Rice, wild, dry	1/4 cup (2.8 oz)	79	160	6	34	0.5	3
Squash, raw, winter (acorn, butternut)	1 cup cubed (4.9 oz)	138	56	1.1	14.6	0.1	2.1
Yam	1 med uncooked (5 oz)	141	180	2.2	39.6	0.2	5.8

Bread, Cereal, Pasta & Grains (Lightly Processed Complex Carbs) X1

Food Item	Qty.	Weight/grams	Calories	Protein	Carbs	Fat	Fiber
Amaranth, whole grain	1/4 cup (1.7 oz)	49	180	7	31	3	7
Bagel, multigrain	1 bagel (3.7 oz)	104	270	11	47	1.5	5
Bagel, plain, whole wheat	1 bagel (3.7 oz)	104	270	12	55	2	1
Bagel, plain, whole wheat high-fiber	1 bagel (3.3 oz)	94	220	11	47	1.5	6
Barley, cracked	1/3 cup (1.6 oz)	46	140	5	33	1	6
Barley, flaked	1/3 cup dry (1.3 oz)	37	110	4	28	1	5
Bread, multigrain	1 slice (1 oz)	28	90	5	19	0.5	4
Bread, multigrain, light (reduced-calorie)	1 slice (.75 oz)	21	60	5	9	1.5	3
Bread, rye	1 slice (1 oz)	28	80	2	215	1.5	1
Bread, rye, light (reduced-calorie)	1 slice (.75 oz)	21	60	5	9	1.5	3
Bread, whole wheat	1 slice (1 oz)	28	100	5	20	1.5	2
Bread, whole wheat, light (reduced-calorie)	1 slice (.75 oz)	21	60	5	8	1.5	3
Bulgur (hot cereal)	1/4 cup dry (1.6 oz)	45	150	5	34	0.5	4
Bulgur (whole grain), dry	1/2 cup (2.5 oz)	71	239	8.6	53.1	0.9	12.8
Cereal, hot, multigrain (oats, rye, barley, triticale, flax)	1/2 cup dry (1.4 oz)	40	140	6	26	2	5
Cereal, hot, multigrain (rye, barley, oats, wheat)	1/2 cup dry (1.4 oz)	40	130	5	29	1	5
Cereal, hot, multigrain (wheat, oats, barley, flax)	1/2 cup dry (1.4 oz)	40	150	6	28	2	6
Couscous, whole wheat, uncooked	1/4 cup dry (1.5 oz)	43	210	8	45	1	7
Cream of buckwheat (hot cereal)	1/4 cup dry (1.8 oz)	50	180	2	41	0	0
Cream of rice (hot cereal)	1/4 cup dry (1.6 oz)	45	170	3	38	0	0
Cream of rye (hot cereal)	1/3 cup dry (1.3 oz)	36	110	5	25	1	5
Cream of wheat (hot cereal)	1/3 cup dry (1.4 oz)	41	120	3.7	24.7	0.7	3.7
Fiber One (boxed cold cereal)	1 cup (2.1 oz)	60	120	4	48	2	26
Granola, honey-sweetened (no sugar added)	1/2 cup (1.9 oz)	55	250	6	31	12	4

Food Item	Qty.	Weight/grams	Calories	Protein	Carbs	Fat	Fiber
Granola, low-fat (no sugar added)	1/2 cup (1.7 oz)	49	186	4	39	2.5	3
Grits, corn (hot cereal)	1/4 cup dry (1.3 oz)	37	130	3	29	0.5	2
Kamut (whole grain), dry	1/4 cup (1.6 oz)	45	170	6	35	1	9
Millet (whole grain), dry	1/4 cup (1.6 oz)	45	160	5	30	2	4
Muesli, hot or cold cereal (oats, grains, nuts, and fruit)	1/4 cup dry (1.1 oz)	31	110	4	21	3	4
Muesli, Swiss, unsweetened (oats, grains, fruit, nuts)	1/2 cup dry	57	210	6	41	3	4
Oat bran (hot cereal)	1/2 cup dry (1.4 oz)	40	120	6	23	3	6
Pita, whole wheat	1 large pita (2.1 oz)	60	140	6	27	1.5	5
Pasta, quinoa, uncooked	3/4 cup dry (2 oz)	56	210	10	42	1	7
Pasta, spaghetti, whole wheat, uncooked	3/4 cup dry (2 oz)	56	210	9	40	1.5	5
Pasta, spelt (whole grain), uncooked	3/4 cup dry (2 oz)	56	210	9	42	1	2
Pasta, spinach, uncooked	3/4 cup dry (2 oz)	56	200	7	41	1	2
Pasta, sprouted multigrain, uncooked	3/4 cup dry (2 oz)	56	210	9	39	2	7
Quinoa (whole grain), flakes	1/3 cup dry (1.2 oz)	34	105	3	23	1	2.2
Rice, brown, boil-in-bag (precooked)	1 bag (3.5 oz)	99	347	9.3	76.4	2.3	4.6
Rice, brown, instant (precooked)	1/4 cup dry (1.7 oz)	48	170	4	36	1	2
Rice cakes, brown rice, plain	1 cake (.07 oz)	0.8	70	1	16	0	0
Shredded wheat, spoon size (boxed cold cereal)	1 cup	49	170	6	40	1	6
Tortilla, corn	2 pcs (1.7 oz)	48	120	3	21	4	0
Tortilla, corn, sprouted	2 pcs (1.7 oz)	48	120	3	23	2	2
Tortilla, multigrain, low-fat	1 large (1.4 oz)	40	100	7	13	1	8
Tortilla, spelt	1 large (2 oz)	57	150	5	28	0	3
Tortilla, whole grain, sprouted (Ezekiel)	1 large (2 oz)	57	150	6	24	3.5	5
Tortilla, whole wheat	1 large (1.6 oz)	47	110	4	16	0	2

Dairy Products (Lean Protein & Natural Carbs)

Food Item	Qty.	Weight/grams	Calories	Protein	Carbs	Fat	Fiber
Milk, skim	1 cup (8 fl oz)	-	90	8	12	0	0
Milk, 1% lowfat	1 cup (8 fl oz)	-	100	8	11	2	0
Milk, 2% lowfat	1 cup (8 fl oz)	-	121	8.1	11.7	4.7	0
Cheese, American, nonfat	2 slices (2 oz)	56	60	10	4	0	0

Dairy Products (Lean Protein & Natural Carbs) *(cont.)*

Food Item	Qty.	Weight/grams	Calories	Protein	Carbs	Fat	Fiber
Cheese, cheddar, lowfat, block	2-inch cube (2 oz)	56	120	18	1	2.5	0
Cheese, cheddar, nonfat, shredded	1/2 cup (2 oz)	56	90	16	4	0	0
Cheese, mozzarella, lowfat, shredded	1/2 cup (2 oz)	56	80	18	2	0	0
Cheese, mozzarella, shredded lowfat (part-skim)	1/2 cup (2 oz)	56	160	16	2	9	0
Cheese, Parmesan, nonfat	2 tbsp (0.4 oz)	11	25	3.3	3.3	0	0
Cheese, Swiss, lowfat	2 slices (2 oz)	56	100	15.9	1.9	2.9	0
Cheese, Swiss, nonfat slices	2 oz	56	81	13.5	5.4	0	0
Cottage cheese, nonfat	1/2 cup (4 oz)	113	100	16.2	7.5	0	0
Cottage cheese, 2% lowfat	1/2 cup (4 oz)	113	102	15.5	4.1	2.2	0
Cottage cheese, 1% lowfat	1/2 cup (4 oz)	113	100	17.5	5	1.3	0
Cream cheese, nonfat	3 oz	85	100	16	4	0	0
Sour cream, lowfat	2 tbsp (1.1 oz)	31	31	1	3	2	0
Sour cream, nonfat	2 tbsp (1.1 oz)	31	25	2	4	0	0
Yogurt, fruit, 1% lowfat	1 yogurt (8 oz)	226	143	11.9	16	3.5	0
Yogurt, fruit, lowfat	1 yogurt (8 oz)	226	240	9	47	2	0
Yogurt, fruit, nonfat	1 yogurt (8 oz)	226	200	16	32	0	0
Yogurt, plain, nonfat	1 yogurt (8 oz)	226	110	10	18	0	0

Fruit (Natural Carbs)

Food Item	Qty.	Weight/grams	Calories	Protein	Carbs	Fat	Fiber
Apple	1 med (5.4 oz)	153	80	0.0	22	0	5
Applesauce, unsweetened (no sugar)	1 cup (8.6 oz)	243	100	0.0	26	0	4
Apricots, fresh	3 med (4 oz)	113	60	0.0	11	0	1
Banana	1 med (4.4 oz)	124	110	1.0	29	0	4
Blackberries	1 cup (5.1 oz)	144	74	1.7	29.6	0.3	3.6
Blueberries	1 cup (5.1 oz)	145	82	1.0	20.4	0.6	4
Canteloupe (melon)	1/2 med (3.5 oz)	99	94	2.3	22.3	0.7	2.1
Cherries, pitted	1 cup, 21 pcs (4.9 oz)	139	90	2.0	22	0	3
Clementine	1 med (2.6 oz)	74	35	0.6	8.9	0	1.3
Cranberries	1 cup (3.4 oz)	96	46	0.4	12	0	4
Figs	1 large (2.3 oz)	65	47	0.5	12.3	0.2	2.1

Food Item	Volume or wt (oz)	Weight (g)	Calories	Protein	Carbs	Fat	Fiber
Grapefruit	1/2 large (4.7 oz)	133	53	1.1	13.4	0.2	1.8
Grapes, seedless red or green	20 grapes (3.4 oz)	96	72	0.6	17.8	0.6	0.6
Goji berries (wolfberries), dried	3 tbsp (1 oz)	28	104	4.0	24	1.3	4
Guava	1 med (4 oz)	113	45	0.7	10.7	0.5	5
Honey, raw (not a fruit, but a natural sugar)	1 tbsp (0.7 oz)	60	60	0.0	17	0	0
Honeydew melon	1 cup, cubed (6 oz)	170	60	0.8	15.6	0.2	1
Jelly, all fruit (no refined sugar)	2 tbsp (1.4 oz)	40	80	0	20	0	0
Kiwifruit	2 med (5.2 oz)	147	100	2	24	0	4
Lemon	1 med (3.8 oz)	108	22	1.3	11.6	0	0
Lime	1 med (2.4)	68	20	0	7	0	2
Mango	1/2 med (4.9 oz)	139	70	0	17	0.5	1
Nectarine	1 med (4.9 oz)	139	70	1.0	16	0	2
Orange	1 med (5 oz)	141	65	1.0	16.3	0.3	3.4
Papaya	1/2 med (4.9 oz)	139	70	0.0	19	0	2
Peach	1 med (3.5 oz)	99	40	1.0	10	0	2
Pear	1 med (5.9 oz)	167	100	1.0	25	1	4
Persimmon	1 med (5.9 oz)	167	118	1.0	31.2	0.3	6
Pineapple	1 cup diced (5.5 oz)	156	76	0.6	19.2	0.6	1.8
Plum	2 med (4.7)	133	80	2.0	38	2	4
Pomegranate	1 large (9.7 oz)	275	104	1.5	26.4	0	0.9
Prunes (dried plums)	5 med (1.5 oz)	42	100	1.0	26	0	3
Raisins	1/4 cup (1.4 oz)	40	130	1.0	31	0	2
Raspberries	1 cup (4.3 oz)	122	61	1.2	14.2	0.6	8.2
Strawberries	halved, 1 cup (5.4 oz)	153	46	1.0	10.6	0	3.6
Tangerines	1 med (3.8)	108	50	1.0	15	0.5	3
Watermelon	1 cup diced (5.4 oz)	153	50	1.0	11.4	0.6	0.8

Fibrous Vegetables & Greens (Natural Complex Carbs)

Food Item	Volume or wt (oz)	Weight (g)	Calories	Protein	Carbs	Fat	Fiber
Artichoke, fresh, edible portions	1 med (4.5 oz)	128	60	4.2	13.5	0.2	6.9
Arugula, raw	1 cup (0.8 oz)	6	6	0.6	0.8	0	0.4
Asparagus spears	10 large 7" (6.6 oz)	187	50	4	8	0	4
Beets, raw	1 cup (6 oz)	170	70	2	16	0	4
Bok choy (Chinese cabbage), raw, shredded	1 cup (2.5 oz)	71	10	1	1.6	0.2	0.8

Fibrous Vegetables & Greens (Natural Complex Carbs) *(cont.)*

Food Item	Volume or wt (oz)	Weight (g)	Calories	Protein	Carbs	Fat	Fiber
Broccoli, raw, chopped	1 cup (3.2 oz)	91	44	4.6	7.8	0.4	4.6
Brussels sprouts, raw, chopped	1 cup (3.1 oz)	88	38	3	7.8	0.2	3.6
Cabbage, raw, shredded	1 cup (3.1 oz)	88	18	1	3.8	0.2	1.6
Carrot, raw	1 large 7.5" (2.8 oz)	79	31	0.7	7.3	0.1	2.2
Cauliflower, raw, chopped	1 cup (3.5 oz)	99	26	2	5.2	0.2	2.6
Celery, raw, stalk	1 med 7.5" (1.6 oz)	45	6	0.3	1.5	0.1	0.7
Chard, Swiss, fresh chopped	1 cup (1.3 oz)	85	6	0.6	1.4	0	0.3
Collard greens, raw	2 cups (2.8 oz)	79	25	2	5	0	3
Cucumber, with peel*	1 small (5.6 oz)	158	19	1	3.4	0	1.1
Eggplant, raw	1 cup pieces (3 oz)	85	22	0.8	5	0.2	2
Garlic, fresh	1 clove	5.6	4	0.2	1	0	0.1
Green beans (string or snap beans), raw	1 cup (4 oz)	113	34	2	7.8	0.2	3.8
Jerusalem artichokes	1/2 cup sliced (3 oz)	85	57	1.5	13.1	0	1.2
Kale, raw, chopped	1 cup (2.4 oz)	68	34	2.2	6.8	0.4	1.4
Leeks, raw	1 cup (3.1 oz)	87	64	1.6	14.9	.4	1.8
Lettuce, romaine, loose leaf, chopped	3 cups (6 oz)	170	30	2	4	0	2
Okra, raw, sliced	1 cup (3.5 oz)	99	38	2	7.6	0.2	2.6
Onion, green (scallion), raw, chopped	1 cup (3.5 oz)	99	32	1.8	7.4	0.2	2.6
Onion, white or yellow, raw, chopped	1 cup (5.2 oz)	147	60	1.8	14	0	2.8
Mushrooms, white, raw pieces or slices	1 cup (2.5 oz)	71	18	2	3	0.4	0.8
Parsnips	1 med (4 oz)	113	85	1.4	20.3	0.3	5.5
Peas, green, frozen	1/2 cup (2.8 oz)	79	60	4	11	0	3
Peas, sugar snap or snow, raw*	1 cup (3 oz)	85	35	2	6	0	2
Pepper, bell or sweet, green or red	med or 1/2 cup (4.2 oz)	119	20	0.7	4.8	0.1	1.3
Pepper, yellow, raw	large (6.6 oz)	187	50	1.9	11.8	0.4	1.7
Pumpkin, raw, cubes	1 cup (4.1 oz)	116	30	1.2	7.6	0.2	2
Radishes, raw, sliced	1/2 cup (2 oz)	57	12	0.4	2.1	0.3	0.9
Salsa or picante sauce, tomato	4 tbsp (4 oz)	115	20	0	5	0	0
Shallots	1 tbsp chopped (0.4 oz)	11	7	0.3	1.7	0	0
Spinach, raw, leaves, chopped	1.5 cups (3 oz)	85	40	2	10	0.4	5
Squash, raw, summer, (zucchini, crookneck)	1 cup (3 oz)	85	16	1.4	3.2	0.2	1.4
Squash, raw, winter (acorn, butternut)	1 cup cubed (4.9 oz)	138	56	1.1	14.6	0.1	2.1

Food Item	Qty.	Weight/grams	Calories	Protein	Carbs	Fat	Fiber
Tomato, whole, raw*	1 med (5.2 oz)	147	35	1	7	0	1
Tomato juice	1 cup (8 fl oz)	-	50	2	10	0	2
Tomato paste	2 tbsp (1.2 oz)	34	30	1	7	0	2
Tomato sauce	1 cup (8 fl oz)	226	80	3	16	0	4
Turnips	1 large (6.5 oz)	184	51	1.7	11.8	0.2	3.3
Turnip greens	3 cups (5.7 oz)	161	42	2.4	9.6	0.6	4.2
Vegetable juice	1 cup (8 fl oz)	-	50	2	10	0	2
Water chestnuts	4 (1.3 oz)	37	35	0	8.6	0	1.1
Watercress	1 cup chopped (1.2 oz)	34	4	0.8	0.4	0	0.8

Fats, Oils, Nuts & Seeds

Food Item	Qty.	Weight/grams	Calories	Protein	Carbs	Fat	Fiber
Almonds, raw	1/4 cup (1.2 oz)	34	210	7	7	19	9
Almond butter, natural (unsweetened)	2 tbsp (1.2 oz)	34	120	0	0	14	0
Avocado*	1.1 oz (1 med)	31	165	3	9	15	9
Brazil nuts, shelled	1/4 cup (4.9 oz)	139	240	5	5	12	2
Cashews, raw	1/4 cup (1.2 oz)	34	190	5	11	15	1
Chia seeds	3 tbsp (1 oz)	28	139	4.4	12.4	10.8	10.7
Coconut oil, extra-virgin	1 tbsp	14	125	0	0	14	0
Coconut, fresh shredded	2 tbsp (1 oz)	28	180	2	7	18	5
Essential oil blend (supplement, not for cooking)	1 tbsp	-	134	0	0	14.2	0
Flaxseed oil (supplement, not for cooking)	1 tbsp	-	130	0	0	14	0
Flaxseed, ground	2 tbsp (0.7 oz)	20	93	4	6	6	4.6
Hazelnuts, dried, chopped	1/4 cup (1 oz)	28	182	3.7	4.4	18	1.7
Macadamia nuts, raw	1/4 cup (1.1 oz)	31	230	3	5	24	2
Olives, Greek black, pitted*	2 oz	56	100	0.6	4	8	0
Olives, green, pitted*	2 oz	56	100	0	4	10	0
Olive oil, extra-virgin	1 tbsp	-	120	0	0	13.6	0
Peanuts, raw	1/4 cup (1.2 oz)	34	214	8.6	7.8	18.1	2.9
Peanut butter, natural (no sugar added)	1 tbsp (0.6 oz)	17	95	4	3.5	8	1
Pecans, halves or pieces	1/4 cup (1 oz)	28	190	3	4	20	3
Pistachios	1/4 cup (1 oz)	28	164	5.8	7.1	13.7	3.1
Pumpkin seeds, whole, in shell, roasted	1/2 cup (2.3 oz)	65	142	5.9	17.2	6.2	0

Food Item	Qty.	Weight/grams	Calories	Protein	Carbs	Fat	Fiber
Salad dressing, balsamic vinaigrette with olive oil, light	2 tbsp	-	45	0	2	4	0
Salad dressing, balsamic vinaigrette, nonfat	2 tbsp	-	5	0	2	0	0
Salad dressing, olive oil and vinegar	1 tbsp	-	75	0	0.5	8	0
Sesame butter	1 tbsp (0.6 oz)	17	100	3	3.6	9	0
Sesame paste (tahini)	1 tbsp (0.5 oz)	14	95	4	1.5	9	0.5
Sesame seeds, whole, dried	1/4 cup (5.1 oz)	144	190	6	8	17	4
Sunflower seeds, shelled	1/4 cup (1 oz)	28	170	7	6	15	3
Walnuts	1/4 cup (1.1 oz)	28	200	5	3	20	3

*Botanically, avocados, tomatoes, and other plant foods with seeds are fruits. Leaves, stems, and roots are vegetables. Legally and traditionally, tomatoes, cucumbers, and peapods are thought of as vegetables. Technically, olives are also a fruit but are listed in fats because of their fat content.

Appendix 4

The Body Fat Solution **Menu Plans**

In this section, you'll find seven days of sample menus compatible with the Body Fat Solution nutrition rules. These menus are only examples, so you're not required to follow them to a T if you don't want to. In fact, I encourage you to learn how to put together your own menu plans because no one knows what you like to eat better than you do.

You may need to customize these menus for your personal calorie requirements and your degree of carbohydrate tolerance. Some people do better on both health parameters and body composition by reducing the X-factor carbs—starches, grains, and simple sugars—and by focusing on eating more of the non-starchy vegetables, low-calorie fruits, lean proteins, and healthy fats.

These menu plans are well balanced and moderate in carbs (no extremes of very high or very low carbs), so they give you a great place to start. With this set of seven menus, at five meals/snacks per day, that's thirty-five meals in total. You can easily mix and match these meals to create additional new menus.

With the portion sizes listed, these menus add up to about 2200 calories per day. That's the average ideal calorie level for men to burn fat while maintaining lean muscle.

Women ususally need about 500–600 calories fewer than men (that's about 1500 to 1600 calories per day). If you're female, all you have to do is eat 75 percent of the portions listed. For example, if a meal says 6 ounces of chicken breast, then women would eat about four ounces. If the menu says one and a half cups of shredded wheat cereal, then you'd eat just over one cup. Simple, right?

If the time comes when you have to reduce your calories, the best way to do it is by selectively reducing the X-factor carbs. Leave the serving sizes of lean protein, fibrous (nonstarchy) vegetables, and healthy fats the same. Instead, reduce your portions of the starchy carbs such as pasta, bread, cereal, and even potatoes, rice, and whole grains.

Last but not least, you'll notice that I've included a handful of my favorite recipes in these menus. It would take another book to give you my entire recipe collection, but I'm sure you'll enjoy this small sampler, and you can get more recipes by visiting me online and subscribing to the email newsletter at www.TheBodyFatSolution.com.

Menu 1

Meal 1 (Breakfast)

2 whole omega-3 eggs and 2 egg whites, scrambled
Low-fat cheddar cheese, shredded, ½ cup
Red pepper, chopped, ½ cup
4-grain hot cereal, oats and flax, 1 cup dry

Meal 2 (Mid-morning snack)

Grapes, 2 cups
Whole-wheat pita (6 inch)

Meal 3 (Lunch)

Chili:
    95% lean ground beef, 6 oz
    Kidney beans, canned, ½ cup
    Chopped garlic and chili powder, to taste

Meal 4 (Mid-afternoon snack)

Nonfat yogurt with fruit
Raw almonds, 20

Meal 5 (Dinner)

99% lean ground turkey, 4 oz
Whole-wheat pasta spirals, 1 cup dry (approx. 2 cups cooked)
Pasta sauce, light tomato and basil, 4.4 oz

Menu #2

Meal 1 (Breakfast)

Whole-wheat bagel, 3.7 oz
Nonfat cream cheese, 3 oz
Raspberries, 1 cup
Nonfat milk, 1 cup

Meal 2 (Mid-morning snack)

1 pear, medium
Celery, 2 stalks
Natural peanut butter, 2 tbsp

Meal 3 (Lunch)

Sprouted wheat bread, 2 slices
Tuna fish, 1 can
Lettuce, tomato, and onion
Reduced-calorie omega-3 mayonnaise, 2 tbsp
Dash of pepper and sea salt

Meal 4 (Mid-afternoon snack)

Low-fat cottage cheese, 1 cup
Sunflower seeds, 2 tbsp
1 peach, large

Meal 5 (Dinner)

Grilled chicken breast, 6 oz
1 baked potato, medium, 7 oz
Steamed spinach, 8 oz
Olive oil, 1 tbsp

Menu #3

Meal 1 (Breakfast)

1 orange, medium, sliced
Greek omelet:
    1 whole omega-3 egg
    3 egg whites
    Chopped spinach, 1½ cups
    Low-fat feta cheese, ¼ cup
    8 Greek black or kalamata olives

Meal 2 (Mid-morning snack)

Nonfat yogurt with fruit, 6 oz
Ground flaxseed (mixed in yogurt)
1 banana, medium

Meal 3 (Lunch)

Tuna, chunk light, 6 oz
Sprouted wheat bread, 2 slices
Hummus (chick pea spread)
1 cucumber, small, sliced

Meal 4 (Mid-afternoon snack)

Low-fat cottage cheese, 1 cup
1 peach, medium, sliced

Meal 5 (Dinner)

Grilled chicken breast, 6 oz
Brown rice, 1 cup
Oriental mixed vegetables, 8 oz
Light soy sauce or Braggs liquid aminos

Menu #4

Meal 1 (Breakfast)

1 orange, medium, sliced
4-veggie omelet or scramble:
    2 whole omega-3 eggs and 2 egg whites
    Mushrooms, onions, tomatoes, green pepper, ½ cup each
    Low-fat (part-skim) mozzarella cheese, ½ cup
    Add your favorite spices to taste

Meal 2 (Mid-morning snack)

Chocolate protein powder, 2 scoops
1 banana, medium
Strawberries, sliced, 1 cup

Meal 3 (Lunch)

Low-fat whole-wheat tortilla
Roasted turkey breast, thin-sliced, 4 oz
4 tomato slices
Lettuce, 1½ cups

Meal 4 (Mid-afternoon snack)

Sardines, canned in olive oil
100% whole-wheat crackers

Meal 5 (Dinner)

Grilled codfish, 6 oz
Baked yam, 6 oz
Mixed green salad:
    Romaine lettuce, 2 cups
    ½ cucumber, medium, sliced
    ½ green pepper, medium, sliced
    1 avocado, medium, sliced
    Light balsamic vinaigrette dressing, 2 tbsp

Meal 1 (Breakfast)

Peach French toast:
    Whole-wheat bread, 2 slices
    Nonfat milk, 1 cup
    Vanilla protein powder, 1 scoop
    Cinnamon, 2 tsp
    Sliced peaches, water-packed, ½ cup

Whisk ingredients, dip bread in milk mixture, cook on skillet 3–4 minutes, top with peaches.

Meal 2 (Mid-morning snack)

Salmon salad pita sandwich:
    Whole-wheat pita, (6 inch)
    Reduced-calorie omega-3 mayonnaise, 1 tbsp
    Chopped onion, ½ cup
    Celery, finely chopped, ¼ cup
    Lemon juice, 2 tbsp
    Dill weed and black pepper, to taste

Meal 3 (Lunch)

Tomato vegetable soup, 1½ cups
Barley, cooked, 1 cup
Low-fat mozzarella cheese, shredded, 1 oz
Tilapia fish, 5 oz

Meal 4 (Mid-afternoon snack)

1 apple, medium
Nonfat fruit yougurt

Meal 5 (Dinner)

Grilled chicken breast, 6 oz
Steamed carrots, 1 cup
Brown rice, cooked, 1 cup

Menu #6

Meal 1 (Breakfast)

Shredded wheat cereal, 1½ cups
Skim milk, 1½ cups
Blueberries, 1 cup

Meal 2 (Mid-morning snack)

Apple-cinnamon oatmeal pancake (a "portable meal"):
   1 whole omega-3 egg
   3 egg whites
   Old-fashioned oatmeal, ¾ cup
   Vanilla protein powder, 1 scoop
   Chopped apple, ½ cup
   Cinnamon, 2 tsp

Mix all ingredients in bowl and cook on fry pan or griddle.

Meal 3 (Lunch)

Grilled chicken breast, 6 oz
1 baked potato, medium
Steamed broccoli, 2 cups

Meal 4 (Mid-afternoon snack)

High-protein meal replacement shake mixed in water, 1 packet

Meal 5 (Dinner)

Beefy Spanish rice:
    Long-grain brown rice, 1 cup
    95% lean ground beef, 6 oz
    Diced tomatoes, canned, 7.5 oz
    Tomato paste, 1 tbsp
    Thyme, black pepper, 2 tsp each
    Worcestershire sauce, 1 tbsp
    Tabasco sauce, 1–2 tsp
    Garlic powder, to taste

Menu #7

Meal 1 (Breakfast)

1 grapefruit, large
Rich and creamy vanilla oatmeal pancakes:
    Old-fashioned oatmeal, 1 cup
    Nonfat cottage cheese, ¾ cup
    4 egg whites

Vanilla protein powder, 1 scoop
Cinnamon, nutmeg, vanilla extract, 1 tsp each

Mix all ingredients in bowl and cook on fry pan or griddle. Makes 2 pancakes.

Meal 2 (Mid-morning snack)

High-protein yogurt:
  Nonfat vanilla yougurt, 6 oz
  Vanilla protein powder, 1 scoop

Meal 3 (Lunch)

Broiled salmon, 5 oz
Steamed asparagus, 10 spears
Brown rice, 1 cup

Meal 4 (Mid-afternoon snack)

Raw almonds, ¼ cup
10 baby carrots, medium

Meal 5 (Dinner)

Grilled top round steak, grass-fed beef, 4 oz
Steamed green beans, 2 cups
1 baked sweet potato, medium